The Zito Trust

THE INSTITUTE OF MENTAL HEALTH LAW

Learning The Lessons

2nd Edition: July 1996

Mental Health Inquiry Reports published in England and Wales between 1969 and 1996 and their recommendations for improving practice.

Compiled by Dave Sheppard
(Director of The Institute of Mental Health Law)
Published by The Zito Trust
ISBN 1 900252 05 8

First published in 1995 by The Zito Trust
Second Edition published in 1996 by The Zito Trust

The Zito Trust is grateful to the authorities concerned for permission to reproduce copyright material. Crown copyright is reproduced with the permission of the Controller of HMSO.
Permission to reproduce material from *The Case of Jason Mitchell: Report of the Independent Panel of Inquiry* and *The Falling Shadow: One Patient's Mental Health Care 1978-1993* is gratefully received from Gerald Duckworth and Company Ltd.

The Zito Trust is grateful to Lundbeck Limited for their sponsorship of this edition of *Learning The Lessons*.

The Zito Trust PO Box 265 London WC2H 9JD Tel: 0171 240 8422
Registered Charity No 1043754

The zito Trust

The Zito Trust was established in July 1994 and is a registered charity (no.1043754). It was set up after the publication of *The Report of the Inquiry into the Care and Treatment of Christopher Clunis* (HMSO, February 1994) which inquired into the circumstances surrounding Jonathan Zito's death at Finsbury Park tube station in December 1992. Jonathan's widow, Jayne Zito, is a founding director, along with Michael Howlett who came from the Special Hospitals Service Authority. The Zito Trust quickly became established as the leading campaigning mental health charity in the field of community care for the severely mentally ill. In providing a comprehensive support service for the victims of the failures of community care, the Trust is in a unique position to raise awareness about the central problems with the policy, and to make comprehensive recommendations for improvements in the way community care services are delivered. In January 1995, The Zito Trust published the first edition of *Learning The Lessons* by Dave Sheppard. This publication brought together for the first time the main mental health inquiry reports published between 1969 and 1994, and grouped the principal recommendations under multi-disciplinary headings. *Learning The Lessons* quickly became the leading publication in this field and has been used by practitioners in mental health and personal social services throughout the country and abroad. It has become an essential training resource for all the disciplines and agencies involved in the delivery of mental health services, particularly in the context of community care. It is also an important historical document.

In addition to these activities, both Jayne Zito and Michael Howlett are actively involved in speaking about these issues and the work of the Trust at conferences, seminars and workshops throughout the country. The Trust is regularly called upon by the media to comment on inquiries and Government policy. Because of the importance of this area of mental health, the Trust has very quickly gained the respect of practitioners from all disciplines in this field, as well as from the media, from policy-makers and the public.

For further information about the work of The Zito Trust, or to offer your support or make a donation, write to:
The Zito Trust, PO Box 265, London WC2H 9JD. Tel/Fax: 0171 240 8422

The Institute of Mental Health Law

Dave Sheppard, Director

Dave Sheppard is a freelance consultant who trains extensively on mental health law and practice throughout England and Wales. He trained as a social worker and worked for nineteen years in the social work departments of both inner city and rural local authorities. He has worked both as a generic and specialist mental health social worker, as well as a manager, in a variety of settings including intake and patch teams, out-of-hours services and psychiatric hospitals. His extensive practical experience includes twelve years as a mental welfare officer and approved social worker. After leaving social work in 1989 he worked for the next three years in the Legal and Parliamentary Unit of MIND.

The Institute of Mental Health Law was formed by Peter Edwards, a Merseyside solicitor, and Dave Sheppard, in 1992, with the aim of promoting a better understanding and awareness of mental health law. The Institute currently provides a comprehensive service (legal consultancy, in-house training, assistance with the formulation of policies and procedures etc.) to several Trusts which provide care to patients with both mental illness and learning disabilities. They have organised a number of highly successful courses and are increasingly being asked to undertake discrete pieces of work for both health and local authorities.

For further information contact The Institute of Mental Health Law, The Stone Cottage, Chapel Corner, Potter Heigham, Norfolk NR29 5LR Phone/Fax: 01692 670772.

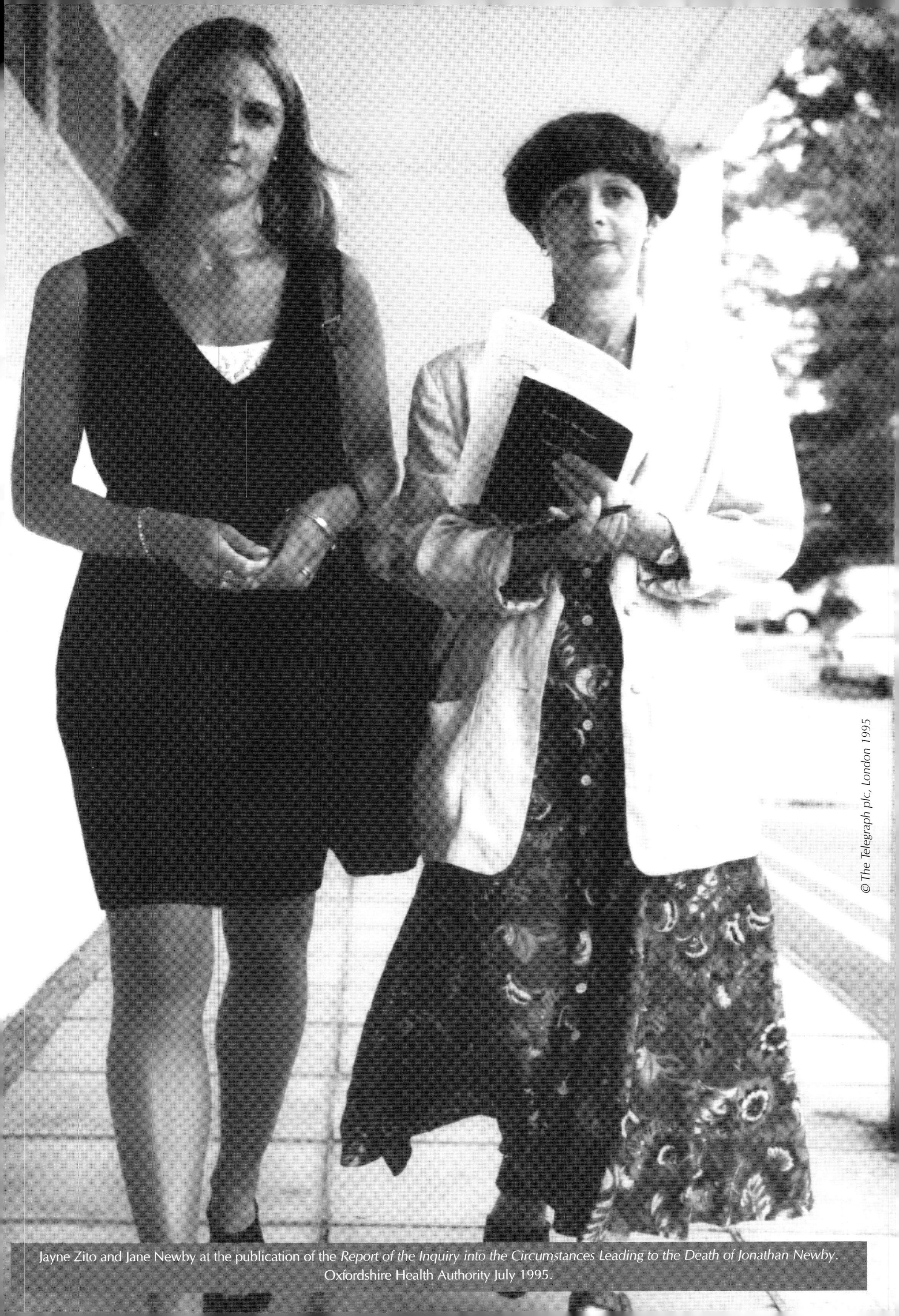

Jayne Zito and Jane Newby at the publication of the *Report of the Inquiry into the Circumstances Leading to the Death of Jonathan Newby.* Oxfordshire Health Authority July 1995.

Contents

FOREWORD

BY

SIR LOUIS BLOM-COOPER QC

In her foreword to the first edition of *Learning The Lessons* Dame Fiona Caldicott, then President of the Royal College of Psychiatrists, welcomed the collation of selected features of the burgeoning inquiry reports after homicides involving mental health patients as providing 'sobering but very enlightening information'. The fact that a second edition is considered necessary within eighteen months of its forerunner appearing is testimony to the unceasing proliferation of inquiries mandated by the Department of Health's circular of May 1994 and to the immense value of Dave Sheppard's unique work as Director of the Institute of Mental Health Law. If there is, sensibly, a desire in many quarters of the mental health system to retrench on the number of inquiries, the sheer accumulation of focused deficiencies in mental health law and practice has had, and is having, a profound impact on official thinking. It cannot be long now before Government orders a thorough-going review of mental health law. The Mental Health Act 1983 reflected a mood in the mental health field that sought to rein in the over-optimistic attitude of psychiatrists. But the additional legalism injected into the 1983 legislation was predicated exclusively upon the notion that doctors required to be controlled in the care and treatment of their patients by medication within the institutional setting of the hospital. *Learning The Lessons* has helped uncover the more pervasive concern about care and treatment in the community. A new legal framework which emphasises that aspect of mental health, with hospitalisation as a back-up to community care, is urgently needed for the 21st century.

The topics selected for noted concern in the second part of the first edition appear fairly comprehensive. The section on Transfer/Leave/Conditional Discharge concentrates on the powers of RMOs and hospital managers. Mental Health Review Tribunals come under scrutiny following the critical remarks in the Jason Mitchell inquiry. The role and functioning of Appropriate Adults described in the Codes of Practice of the Police and Criminal Evidence Act 1984 was a notable omission from the first edition. Dave Sheppard's impressive work elsewhere on that aspect of mental health deserves to find a place in *Learning The Lessons*.*

All this starkly points to a third edition in 1997. Until some of the recurrent defects of the present law and practice are instantly addressed by Government and Parliament, the continuing need for a publication entitled *Learning The Lessons* remains pressing. I commend the second edition to keep all practitioners in mental health up-to-date with what is happening at the coal-face. There is nothing so debilitating of good practice as ignorance of both good and bad practice in the contemporary mental health system.

Sir Louis Blom-Cooper QC

* *The Appropriate Adult : A Review of the Case Law 1988-1995*, Second Edition, June 1996. Available from The Institute of Mental Health Law

INTRODUCTION

JAYNE ZITO and MICHAEL HOWLETT
DIRECTORS of THE ZITO TRUST

Nineteen ninety-five saw the publication of the first edition of *Learning The Lessons* which listed some thirty-nine inquiries and over three hundred recommendations. In the first edition, the author, Dave Sheppard, described his search for earlier inquiries and made reference to what he then thought was the oldest available, which was published in 1632. He has since discovered an even earlier inquiry from 1403, which reported on conditions in Bethlem Hospital. Much of the information relating to the later inquiries came from John Martin's book *Hospitals in Trouble*, published in 1984 and now out of print.

The second edition of *Learning The Lessons* follows the same format as the first. The recommendations are listed chronologically under each of the subject headings, and a recommendation will appear only once - under the heading most suited to it. This, of course, does not mean it might not appear elsewhere.

We are both very grateful to Dave Sheppard for his excellent work in bringing these inquiries together in such a powerful and constructive document.

In the foreword to the first edition of *Learning The Lessons*, published in January 1995, Jayne Zito wrote:

> ***"Other major inquiries are due to report in 1995; there will be more recommendations and, distressingly, it is likely there will be further incidents involving community care patients."***

It is sad to report, with the publication now of the second edition, that we have to include another fifteen independent inquiry reports into homicides involving the mentally disordered. Fourteen of these were published in the last eighteen months. Among the total are *The Falling Shadow*, which inquired into the circumstances surrounding the death of Georgina Robinson at the Edith Morgan Centre in Torbay; also included are Jonathan Newby, who was killed by John Rous at Jacqui Porter House in Oxford in October 1993; and Jason Mitchell, Shaun Armstrong, Nilesh Gadher, Frank Hampshire, Raymond Sinclair, The Woodley Team Report, the Viner Report, the Grey Report, Philip McFadden in Scotland, Brian Doherty in Northern Ireland, and the case of Erhi Inweh who killed volunteer worker Katie Sullivan in a MIND hostel in Kingston-upon-Thames. Katie's mother Sandra Sullivan has campaigned forcefully and passionately for a proper independent inquiry into her daughter's death but has been shabbily treated by the authorities in this respect.

Sadly, too, as we go to press, we have to report that many more independent inquiries are due to publish in the coming months (Anthony Smith, Martin Mursell, Richard Linford, Peter Horrod and others), and our own initial research into the number of homicides committed by mentally disordered people shows (contrary to the stock response on this subject) that the number has increased since the acceleration of the Government's community care policies in 1991 and the current fast-track hospital closure programme. The figures quoted (100 deaths in three years, 34 in three years, one a month, two a month) are confusing because their source - *The Confidential Inquiry into Homicides and Suicides* (the 'Boyd Report') - is confusing, partly because it does not purport to be an epidemiological study. The work on the Confidential Inquiry is now to be carried out at the University of Manchester, under the directorship of Dr Louis Appleby.

We thought hard about adding a question mark to the second edition of *Learning The Lessons*, as in *Learning The Lessons?*, to make the point that since the publication of the seminal *Report of the Inquiry into the Care and Treatment of Christopher Clunis* in February 1994, not much has been learned, with the very important exception that the death of Jonathan Zito in December 1992 was not an isolated incident and that the Government's policy for caring for the severely mentally ill in the community has been shown, in far too many cases, to be a disaster. The evidence contained in the inquiries Dave Sheppard has brought together, in conjunction with the many inquiries still to report, is incontrovertible. For a long time the stock ministerial response was 'a good policy, with some teething problems', or 'responsibility for implementation lies with local authorities'. This kind of evasive response did not fool anyone, certainly not the media, and in February 1996 the Secretary of State for Health stood up in the House of Commons and effectively admitted that the policy was fundamentally flawed, partly by changing its name to 'The Spectrum of Care' - and by introducing a new raft of measures to add to the long list of elastoplast measures, including new legislation (Mental Health (Patients in the Community) Act 1995), that have flowed with telling regularity from central government.

If we sound sceptical it is because we have had too much direct experience and evidence from the operation of our support service at The Zito Trust, and from our contacts on the conference and training circuit throughout the country. Professionals working across all the major disciplines in this field have become increasingly demoralised and frustrated by their inability to do a difficult job in difficult conditions effectively, and by what they perceive as inappropriate and unhelpful paperwork issuing out of central government. The Royal College of Psychiatrists, a relatively conservative body of professionals, recently passed a resolution condemning the current state of mental health services and calling upon the Government to take immediate action. In a follow-up article in the Daily Express (12 July 1996), the College's Registrar, Professor Chris Thompson, describes a deepening crisis largely exacerbated by the Government's refusal to call a moratorium on bed closures. The situation for patients and public alike, says Professor Thompson, 'is dangerous [and] must be resolved as a matter of urgency'. He goes on to call for a major conference to reappraise the entire community care programme.

Such a conference would undoubtedly hear how badly off and unfocused many local mental health services are. These services clearly lack the basic requirements: the finance, planning, training, supervision and the right tools for the job. It goes without saying that community care for the mentally ill is vitally dependent on the right services being in place before beds are closed and patients discharged. The failure of the policy in so many cases is a damning reflection of the almost complete absence of any strategic planning in this area. Effective community care services are complex in their structure, management and costs; they have specialised resource needs and require a completely different set of skills from hospital care. One of the baselines for the consistent delivery of these therapeutic services across the care range is pro-active and efficient communication between all the agencies involved. Or, indeed, any communication. The inter-agency communication which is at the heart of the Care Programme Approach is largely non-existent - but could that be because the Care Programme Approach, which has been an obligation on the authorities since 1991, has still not yet been fully implemented?

It would seem to be a luxury to hope that relatively sophisticated measures like the Care Programme Approach will one day be universally understood and applied when one looks at the dreadful state of the basic services, particularly in the inner cities, and the appalling pressures experienced by professionals, patients, families and informal carers. Just as we are preparing to publish *Learning The Lessons* we read of the Mental Health Act Commission's recent report on St Anne's Hospital in Haringey, where overcrowding has become so acute that patients are forced to sleep on mattresses on the floor, and even in armchairs. These conditions, which may be found in many hospitals throughout the country, must be set in the context of the Department of Health's recently published statistics (Bulletin 1996/10) which show that the number of in-patients formally detained in NHS and private hospitals under the Mental Health Act 1983 between 1989/90 and 1994/95 rose by 55%, from 17,400 to 27,100. Many of these admissions are revolving door patients who have unwittingly become the victims of bed closures, overcrowding and the consequent 'hotbedding' that attempts to alleviate it. Is this approach to treatment one of the hallmarks of a civilised society and one which we can be proud of?

The victim support service we have been offering now at The Zito Trust for the past two years has made us well aware of the problems faced by those caught up in the system. The service we offer is unique in that its focus is exclusively on the problems with community care experienced by families, formal and informal carers, and members of the public. We have received hundreds of calls from people trying to access the basic services, people trying to get through. Our database describes the whole range of community care problems, from homicides to the dangerous lack of understanding and awareness displayed by housing associations, some of them well known. We continue to support and represent the secondary victims of community care homicides - bereaved families whose loved ones we are told were 'in the wrong place at the wrong time'. In our view it was the patient who committed the homicide who was 'in the wrong place at the wrong time'. Too often the severely mentally ill are simply left in what's called the 'community' to deteriorate in situations which make them increasingly vulnerable and at risk of harming themselves and/or other people. Monahan's work on risk assessment, which is far more sophisticated than the convenient excuse that 'the best (or only) predictor of future behaviour is past behaviour', would describe these patients, who have been abandoned by the shortcomings of flawed policies, as approaching the top rung of 'the ladder of dangerousness'. See the *Report of the Inquiry into the Treatment and Care of Raymond Sinclair* (June 1996, at page 66) for further discussion of Monahan's work.

But what of the future of the independent inquiries themselves? Where there is a homicide involving previous contact with the specialist mental health services there must, under Health Service Guidelines (HSG(94)27), Chapter 5 of *Building Bridges*), be an independent inquiry and a published report available to the public. The guidance seems clear on this and yet there is still some confusion (e.g. *The Hampshire Report*) about whether an independent inquiry needs to be held in certain circumstances (Francis Hampshire was an outpatient at the time). This lack of certainty, prevarication in some cases, leads to unnecessary delay which benefits nobody. There are, additionally, cases involving the death of children which raise urgent child protection issues in the context of essential adult mental health considerations which have not gone to independent inquiry (Sharon Dalson, Haringey, 1994; Aidan Kenny, Manchester, 1994), so the process is by no means uniform in its implementation. It is therefore difficult to know at this stage exactly how many independent inquiries there are and how many there should be.

What we do know is that there have been - there still are - so many of these inquiries that a number of commentators in this field feel that it's all gone too far, it costs too much, it no longer serves any purpose, and the system should be scrapped. Indeed the Department of Health is actively working to produce a consultation document on the future management of independent inquiries which may, on the one hand, be tantamount to moving the goalposts and yet which could, on the other hand, be viewed as a defensive response to the Government's embarrassment about these unnecessary and tragic deaths. We are convinced that independent inquiries should continue to be held, largely because the internal inquiries are the exact opposite of independent, they are not sufficiently investigative and few people outside the organisation concerned get to read them.

That there are so many independent inquiries of a public nature is a statement per se of the terrifying scale of the problem. It is because there continue to be so many failures, many of which are quite properly highlighted by the press. Each inquiry sets out to 'learn the lessons' from the particular tragedy so that other tragedies can be prevented. This worthy ambition has a hollow ring about it now. It seems that every authority in the country would need to have its homicide, perhaps more than one, followed by its inquiry, followed by its action plan ('many of the recommendations made in the report have already been implemented' is a typical response from the chief executive of the moment) before there is any chance of any lesson being learned at the local level. Surely this is because there is no mechanism contained in the independent inquiry process - or the guidance for it - for the panel, or anyone else, to return to the authority concerned some six or twelve months after the report has been published to monitor the progress that has really been made with the implementation of the recommendations. To our knowledge, the only case where this has happened is Oxfordshire Health Authority, following the publication of the Jonathan Newby report and as a result of a specific and public request from Jayne Zito at the publication of the report that the Health Authority undertake to follow up the work of the inquiry team. A clear recommendation was made in the Jason Mitchell inquiry report, where Suffolk Health were asked to invite :

> ***'the members of the Inquiry Panel to reconvene, in private, within six months of publication of this report, to consider the responses, both official and unofficial, to the recommendations; and to report activity . . . early in 1997.'***

Suffolk Health instantly accepted the recommendation. The panel is due to reconvene in November 1996 and will publish its report in 1997.

Surely this is the most constructive way forward from these inquiries - but will such a recommendation be uniformly adopted?

We would like to see the NHS Executive implement Recommendation 12 in the *Report of the Inquiry into the Treatment and Care of Raymond Sinclair* (West Kent, June 1996)

(i) A panel should be set up to supervise inquiries commissioned under Health Service Guidelines HSG(94)27.

(ii) The panel should be responsible for creating a register of those suitably qualified, both professionally and in their interpersonal skills, to sit on such inquiries.

(iii) It should also publish a recommended form of procedure and additional guidance designed to reduce delay and the stress caused to witnesses, particularly the relatives of the deceased and other victims, and to encourage cost-effectiveness.

In addition, we would like to see measures implemented for disseminating each inquiry report to all agencies and authorities responsible for the purchase and provision of mental health services in England and Wales and, further, measures for ensuring that members of the central panel described above return to the authorities concerned to monitor their progress in improving practice according to the recommendations specific to them and those from the other published inquiries which have currency on a national basis. Both the Newby and Mitchell inquiry reports were disseminated by their respective commissioning authorities to every health authority and provider trust in the country.

The view about independent inquiries into failures by mental health services, that they are counter-productive, that they lead to defensive practices and that, on occasions, they scapegoat individual practitioners, has been well aired. In *Inquiries after Homicide*, published by Duckworth (1996), in conjunction with the Jason Mitchell report, David Carson suggests that inquiries should also be concerned about their moral responsibilities, that they should, inter alia:

> ***'...make it plain to their readers what the public legitimately can and cannot expect from mental health care services. They should be explicit about the legislative restrictions on clinicians, including the fact that public safety is not the exclusive criterion for decision-making. They should emphasise that community care, particularly where there are no grounds for detention, is not just a policy but a legal duty. They should be explicit in emphasising that mental health services cannot be provided on a no-risk basis. They should keep repeating what we know about***

homicides by people with mental disorders, in particular that the risk of violence to others is grossly exaggerated and that it is the apparent randomness in choice of victim, in several cases, that causes much of the public fear.' (page 143)

In the same publication Nigel Eastman claims the independent inquiry policy in community care homicides is essentially driven by political purposes. He points to the absence of a 'proper level of risk of mentally disordered homicide compared with other medical mishaps' and goes on to recommend the abolition of mandatory inquiries.

On this question of risk, we at The Zito Trust take issue with the implied notion that you can do little more than predict future behaviour by looking at past behaviour, with the additional implication that you can never predict violent acts or homicides and hardly ever prevent them. Our view is that this is the application and endorsement of poor working practices which quickly become the cultural mean for services which are not only short-staffed, under-resourced and traditionally marginalised but which seem to be constantly undergoing reorganisation at the time of the incident taking place. It is almost as if the only way for demoralised practitioners to cope with increased (and more dangerous) caseloads is to go on a course, go sick, undergo organisational change, or even, in a number of cases, *go on holiday*. These are undoubtedly well documented defensive techniques by the individual and/or the organisation. What they are not is acceptable methodologies for the process of making decisions about the clinical management of patients in forensic psychiatry. The Sinclair Inquiry (at page 66) makes this point very well:

'[b]oth recent research findings and properly deployed intuition enable clinicians nowadays to go well beyond the limitations of the oft-repeated adage "nothing predicts violence like previous violence".'

Proper tools are available to do the job far better than it is being done at the moment. There is no excuse for not using these tools. Mistakes in this field cost lives. That is what the independent inquiries demonstrate loud and clear. We should continue to have access to this message whatever the cost or inconvenience to those who don't want to hear it.

An additional point sometimes raised is that more people die on the roads, or through alcohol or drug abuse, so why are there not mandatory inquiries investigating these deaths? We answered this point in a letter to the *Health Service Journal* in March 1996 where we wrote:

'How can you equate the risk of driving a car with the appalling mismanagement of Christopher Clunis' care in the community and the brutal attack on Jonathan Zito, a complete stranger, which followed it? It would have to be a rust bucket of a car, with three wheels and blinkers for headlights.'

In the same issue there was a letter from Professor Elaine Murphy, former vice-chair of the Mental Health Act Commission, who drew attention to the importance of inquiries from the family's perspective. Too often, in our experience, the bereaved family is doubly victimised, first by the homicide itself, secondly by a process that should help them but which often leaves them feeling isolated and uncared for. In Professor Murphy's words:

'..inquiries are not set up only to prevent recurrences. They also provide explanations and insight for bereaved relatives and, in the case of homicides, also for the family of the mentally ill person who often feel abandoned and let down by the services. As public servants, surely managers and clinicians must be ready to have their practice scrutinised and should demonstrate a positive willingness to be criticised when criticism is justified?'

A similar point is made by Professor Paul Rock in *Inquiries After Homicide*.

An inquiry should, therefore, be conducted in a uniform manner, with the bereaved family uppermost in its consideration and modus operandi. The central panel recommended by the Sinclair inquiry, and endorsed by The Zito Trust, would place the family firmly on the agenda, not only to allow them to give evidence as a matter of course but also to ensure that they are respected and nurtured throughout the inquiry process as befits people who have been bereaved by violence. This includes the basic courtesies of having information in advance (not having to seek it out), being interviewed by the whole panel, not simply by a few members of it, and having at the end of the inquiry a published report of good quality which they can read before the official publication date. Some of the reports we have seen are a disgrace and an insult to people who have lost loved ones and have clearly been done on the cheap.

Finally, in speaking of the secondary victims, it is noteworthy that the Home Secretary's recent proposals to pilot 'victim impact statements' in six police force areas exclude such statements from those bereaved by homicide. We see this as a serious lapse and endorse the recommendation to this effect made by the Parliamentary All Party Penal Affairs Group in their report *Increasing The Rights of Victims of Crime* (July 1996). The more the system gets to hear about the full impact of what has happened - particularly in cases of homicide - and what people think should happen next, the better. Listen to how people feel and respect their views. They have an important story to tell.

The irony is that an alarming number of published inquiry reports reveal that had the family and/or those close to the family been listened to by professionals in the first place, there is every chance the homicide would not have taken place.

While we recognise that The Zito Trust has a particular focus on homicides and the inquiries which follow them, we do not underestimate the importance of reducing the rate of suicides in this country. Chapter 5 of the Department of Health's *Building Bridges* states that lessons need to be learned from the required local audit of suicides and undetermined deaths of mentally ill people. It is difficult, however, to know just how lessons can be learned when these local audits are not disseminated nationally, are not even in the public domain. The entire system needs to have access to the information in order to apply the lessons. We wonder whether this kind of local audit is indeed the future destination for homicide inquiries. Such a move would be a retrograde step.

The purpose in bringing inquiries together under one roof in *Learning The Lessons* is to enable practitioners and others to use the valuable tools collected here. With the appropriate willpower, belief and effort, the numerous recommendations brought together can be, must be, taken on board and implemented. Otherwise the exercise we are engaged in is an arid one, without much purpose beyond the merely historical one of creating an archive. We do not believe this is the fundamental purpose of *Learning The Lessons*, but it is now for others to make the next move.

Jayne Zito, Michael Howlett

Directors, The Zito Trust
London, July 1996

SUMMARY OF EVENTS LEADING TO THE SETTING UP OF INQUIRIES BETWEEN 1985 - 1996 AND THEIR TERMS OF REFERENCE

1996

REPORT OF THE INQUIRY INTO THE TREATMENT AND CARE OF RAYMOND SINCLAIR

Richard Lingham, Dr Julian Candy and John Bray

Raymond Sinclair was born in 1961. He was informally admitted to Joyce Green Hospital in April 1994 when an initial diagnosis of a "hypomanic episode" was made. He was returned to the ward by the police on three occasions (once under s.136, Mental Health Act 1983). He was discharged in June 1994 but readmitted for one week in August 1994 after he threatened his brother with a bread knife. He returned to live with his mother in her one bedroomed flat. He was seen as an out-patient and supported by Community Psychiatric Nurses and a Social Worker.

On 3rd November 1994, Raymond Sinclair fatally stabbed his mother, Mary Povey, fifteen times with a vegetable knife. On 10th November 1995 he was convicted of manslaughter and detained in Broadmoor Hospital under ss.37/41, Mental Health Act 1983.

The terms of reference of the Inquiry, set up in December 1995, were to:

▲ examine all the circumstances surrounding the treatment and care of Raymond Sinclair by the mental health services, in particular:

(i) the quality and scope of his health care, social care and risk assessments;

(ii) the appropriateness of his hospital treatment and in patient care and subsequent support, supervision and after care in the community, in respect of:

a) his assessed health and social care needs;

b) his assessed risk of potential harm to himself or others;

c) any previous psychiatric history;

d) the number and nature of any previous court convictions;

(iii) the extent to which his care corresponded to statutory obligations; relevant guidance from the Department of Health (including the Care Programme Approach, discharge guidance and local operational policies);

(iv) the extent to which his prescribed care plans were:

a) effectively delivered, and

b) complied with by Raymond Sinclair;

(v) the history of Raymond Sinclair's medication and compliance with the regimes.

▲ examine the adequacy of the collaboration and communication between:

(i) the agencies (Thameslink Healthcare Services NHS Trust and Kent SSD) involved in the care of Raymond Sinclair or in the provision of services to him, and

(ii) the statutory agencies and his family.

▲ prepare a report and make recommendations to West Kent Health Authority and Kent SSD.

The report was published in June 1996 by West Kent Health Authority, Preston Hall, Aylesford, Kent ME20 7NJ (01622-710161).

THE REPORT OF THE INQUIRY INTO THE CARE AND TREATMENT OF SHAUN ARMSTRONG

Mr C Freeman, Mr A Brown, Dr D Dunleavy, Mr F Graham

Shaun Armstrong was born in 1962. He had received inpatient care on three different wards at Hartlepool General Hospital during his five informal admissions between March 1992 and June 1993. He subsequently attended three out-patient appointments but failed his appointment on 5th May 1994. On the afternoon of 30th June 1994 Rose (Rosie) Palmer aged almost four years left her home in Hartlepool to buy an ice cream. On the 3rd July 1994 her body was found by the Police in a plastic bag at the home of Shaun Armstrong who lived approximately fifty yards away. Rosie had been raped, otherwise sexually abused and her body had been mutilated following her death. Shaun Armstrong was arrested and on the 22nd July 1995 at Leeds Crown Court. He pleaded guilty to murder and was sentenced to life imprisonment. In passing sentence, the Judge stated that Shaun Armstrong was a severely disordered personality but had been fully responsible for his actions at the time of the murder. He is currently detained at Wakefield Prison.

The terms of reference of the Inquiry, set up in August 1995, were to:

- establish the care that Shaun Anthony Armstrong was receiving at the time of the incident including the history of his medication and compliance with regimes;
- establish the suitability of such care in view of the patient's history and assessed health, social care needs, any previous psychiatric history or court convictions;
- establish the adequacy of the assessment of the patient's risk to himself and others;
- establish compliance or otherwise with statutory obligations, relevant guidance from the Department of Health and local policies;
- establish the exercise of professional judgement;
- establish the adequacy of the care plan and Shaun Anthony Armstrong's compliance with it;
- establish the adequacy of monitoring arrangements by key worker;
- establish the adequacy of communication by health staff and use of liaison arrangements between Health Agencies and between Health and other agencies;
- prepare a report and make recommendations to Tees District Health Authority.

The report was published in June 1996 by Tees Health Authority, Poole House, Stokesley Rd, Nunthorpe, Middlesborough TS7 0NJ (01642 - 320000) - price £10. Cheque made payable to *HM Paymaster General* to accompany order.

THE HAMPSHIRE REPORT: REPORT OF THE INDEPENDENT INQUIRY TEAM INTO THE CARE AND TREATMENT OF FRANCIS HAMPSHIRE

Jane Mishcon, Dr Donald Dick, Ian Milne, Paul Beard and Jane Mackay

Frank Hampshire was born in 1933 and he married Catherine in 1957. They were both teachers. There was no overtly serious problem with his mental health until about 1983/4. In June 1985 he was referred by his GP to the psychiatric services at Goodmayes Hospital. Over the next nine years he was admitted to hospital on two occasions (once under s.2, Mental Health Act 1983). He also was seen as an outpatient and was visited by a Community Psychiatric Nurse.

At about midnight on 31st May 1994, Frank Hampshire killed his wife, aged 62, in a frenzied attack, stabbing her over 300 times in the head and neck. On 5th December 1994, at the Central Criminal Court, his plea of guilty to manslaughter on the grounds of diminished responsibility was accepted and he was detained in Rampton Hospital under ss.37/41, Mental Health Act 1983.

Although Frank Hampshire was an outpatient at the time of his wife's death, there was no internal inquiry. Furthermore, there was confusion as to whether or not there was a requirement to hold an independent inquiry, as a result of which this inquiry was not set up until the end of 1995.

The terms of reference of the Inquiry were to:

- investigate all the circumstances surrounding the treatment and care of Frank Hampshire by the Mental Health Services, in particular:

  (i) the quality and scope of his health and social care and risk assessment.

  (ii) the appropriateness of his treatment, care and supervision in respect of:
  a) his assessed health and social care needs;
  b) the assessed risk of harm to himself and others;
  c) his psychiatric history;
  d) the relevance of court convictions (if any).

  (iii) the professional and in service training of those involved in his care and treatment or in the provision of services to him.

  (iv) the extent to which his care and treatment corresponded to the relevant statutory obligations, Department of Health guidelines, and local policies and procedures.

  (v) the extent to which his care and treatment plans were effectively drawn up, communicated and delivered.

  (vi) the history of his compliance with treatment plans and advice of those responsible for his care.

  (vii) to evaluate the adequacy of the co-ordination and communication between the agencies (Redbridge Health Care NHS Trust, his GP and any other agencies) who were or who might appropriately have been involved in his care and how effectively they worked jointly in that care.

- prepare a report and make recommendations to Redbridge & Waltham Forest Health Authority.

The report was published in May 1996 by Redbridge and Waltham Forest Health Authority, West Wing, 713 Eastern Avenue, Ilford, Essex IG2 7SJ (0181-518-2299).

REPORT OF THE INDEPENDENT INQUIRY TEAM INTO THE CARE AND TREATMENT OF NILESH GADHER

His Honour John Main QC, Dr John Wilkins, David Pope and Steve Manikon

Nilesh Gadher was born in 1958. He qualified as a pharmacist and worked in this capacity for about five years. He was first referred to a psychiatrist in 1984 when a diagnosis of paranoid schizophrenia was made. In May 1985 he was charged with forging prescriptions and placed on probation. The following year he was struck off the Pharmaceutical Register. He was admitted to hospital on three occasions under the provisions of the Mental Health Act 1983.

On 6th September 1994 Nilesh Gadher ran over and killed Sanita Kaura, aged 27, a complete stranger. He was found unfit to plead at the Old Bailey on 21st July 1995 and sent to a special hospital.

The terms of reference of the Inquiry were to:

- examine all the circumstances surrounding the treatment and care of Nilesh Gadher by the mental health services, in particular the appropriateness of his treatment, care and supervision in respect of:
  - a) his assessed health and social care needs;
  - b) his assessed risk of potential harm to himself or others;
  - c) any previous psychiatric history;
  - d) the number and nature of any previous court convictions.

- examine the extent to which his care corresponded to statutory obligations, particularly the Mental Health Act 1983; relevant guidance from the Department of Health (including the Care Programme Approach, Supervision Registers, discharge guidance HSG(94)27); and local operational policies.

- examine the extent to which his prescribed care plans including medication were:
  a) effectively delivered; b) complied with;

- examine the adequacy of the collaboration and communications between:
  The agencies (Hounslow and Spelthorne Community and Mental Health NHS Trust, Hounslow Social Services, the General Practitioner and the Star Centre) involved in the care of Nilesh Gadher or in the provision of services to him, and the statutory agencies and his family;

- consider the overall standard of care arrangements offered and the relationship between these arrangements and the events of 6th September 1994;

- prepare a report and make recommendations to Ealing, Hammersmith and Hounslow Health Authority and the London Borough of Hounslow.

The report was published in April 1996 and is available from Ealing, Hammersmith and Hounslow Health Authority, 1 Armstong Way, Southall, UB2 4SA (0181-893-0303).

THE VINER REPORT: THE REPORT OF THE INDEPENDENT INQUIRY INTO THE CIRCUMSTANCES SURROUNDING THE DEATHS OF ROBERT AND MURIEL VINER

Anthony Harbour, Dr John Brunning, Linda Bolter and Helen Hally

Robert Viner was born in 1953. He first received treatment for mental illness in 1971. In 1976 he moved to Dorset to live with his mother. Apart from two brief inpatient admissions as an informal patient in 1981 and 1982 he lived with and was cared for by his mother. From 1976 onwards he had contact with the mental health services in Dorset - the degree and nature of this contact varied over the years. On the 19th April 1995, a community psychiatric nurse visited and, because of the deteriorating situation, contacted a psychiatrist and requested that the offer of a hospital bed be made to Robert Viner to give his mother a break. Later that day, while sitting in an armchair in her living room, Muriel Viner, aged 76, received more than twelve blows to the head from a heavy metal disc which was found on the floor near her body. Robert Viner died some time later from an overdose of drugs. His body was found in the bath upstairs.

The terms of reference of the Inquiry were to:

- examine all the circumstances surrounding the treatment and care of Robert Viner by the Mental Health and Social Services, in particular:

  the quality and scope of his health, social care and risk assessments;

  the suitability of his treatment, care and supervision in respect of:
  his assessed health and social care needs;
  his assessed risk of potential harm to himself or others;
  any previous psychiatric history;
  the number and nature of any previous court convictions;

  the extent to which his care corresponded to statutory obligations; relevant guidance from the Department of Health; and local operational policies;

  the extent to which his prescribed care plan was:
  effectively delivered;
  complied with by Robert Viner;
  monitored by the Key Worker;

  the history of Robert Viner's medication and compliance with that regime;

- consider the adequacy of the training in the assessment of risk of all the mental health care staff involved in Robert Viner's care;

- examine the adequacy of the collaboration and communication between:
  the agencies (Dorset HealthCare NHS Trust and Dorset Social Services, Knightstone and other Housing Agencies and GP), involved in the care of Robert Viner, or in the provision of services to him, and the statutory agencies, Robert Viner's GP and Muriel Viner;

- consider the adequacy of the support given to Muriel Viner by the mental health care services;

- review recommendations of the internal inquiry and advise whether any additions or amendments to their recommendations are necessary;
- consider such other matters relating to the said matters as the public interest may require;
- prepare a report and make recommendations to Dorset Health Commission.

The report was published in March 1996 by Dorset Health Commission, Victoria House, Princes Rd, Ferndown, Dorset BH22 9JR (01202-893000) - price £14. Cheque, made payable to *Dorset Health Authority,* to accompany order.

THE CASE OF JASON MITCHELL: REPORT OF THE INDEPENDENT PANEL OF INQUIRY

Sir Louis Blom-Cooper QC, Dr Adrian Grounds, Pat Guinan, Anne Parker and Michael Taylor

Jason Mitchell was born in 1970. He was seen by a psychiatrist on a number of occasions whilst he was serving a period of 2 years' youth custody for robbery and other offences. In 1990 he attacked a cleaner at St Barnabas Church, Epsom and was charged with attempted murder and other offences. He subsequently pleaded guilt at the Central Criminal Court to common assault and possession of offensive weapons (two knives). He was made the subject of a hospital order with restrictions (ss.37/41, Mental Health Act 1983). In May 1994 he moved to shared accommodation run by MIND in Felixtowe but, following disruptive behaviour, was readmitted to Easton House as an informal patient. On 9th December 1994 he left and failed to return and on 20th December 1994 he was arrested following the discovery by police of the bodies of his father, aged 54, and neighbours Arthur and Shirley Wilson, both aged 65. In July 1995, Jason Mitchell was sentenced to three terms of life imprisonment for manslaughter on the grounds of diminished responsibility. On 9th May 1996 he successfully appealed and was instead made the subject of a hospital order with restrictions (ss.37/41, Mental Health Act 1983).

The terms of reference of the Inquiry, set up in May 1995 were to:

- examine and assess the quality of treatment and continuing care of Jason Mitchell, leading up to his absence from Easton House, St Clement's Hospital, Ipswich on 9th December 1994, in particular the appropriateness of such care and treatment, having regard to:

    his socio-medical history, including any previous psychiatric treatment;

    the index offence of 8th February 1990 leading up to the conviction at the Central Criminal Court on 10th September 1990 and any other relevant criminal events;

    the deferred conditional discharge by the Mental Health Review Tribunal in September 1991 plus the similar order made by the Mental Health Review Tribunal on 6th April 1993;

    his mental health while at West Park Hospital, 1991-93;

    assessments from time to time of risk of harm to himself and others;

any indications of deterioration in mental health immediately prior to 9th December 1994;

any behaviour of an unusual nature during the period of conditional discharge in 1991 and after-care supervision, 1991-94;

the extent to which Jason Mitchell's mental health care matched the statutory obligation, relevant guidance from the Department of Health, discharge guidance and local operational policies;

the extent to which any prescribed care plan for Jason Mitchell was effectively delivered to him and complied with;

the history both of prescribed medication and of the use of illegal drugs;

- inquire into the circumstances leading up to and surrounding Jason Mitchell's continued absence from Easton House, from 9th - 20th December 1994, in particular, to examine the adequacy of local arrangements for dealing with patients who absent themselves from hospital, the effectiveness and efficacy of such arrangements and the exercise of individual responsibilities, including a review of the aftermath of Jason Mitchell's absconding in February/March 1994;

- examine the adequacy and appropriateness of inter-agency arrangements for collaboration among, and communication between the relevant agencies - Suffolk Health Authority; East Suffolk Local Health Services NHS Trust; Suffolk Police Authority; C3 Division of the Home Office; Suffolk County Council Social Services Department; Suffolk Coastal District Council Housing Department; and East Suffolk MIND - in the provision of care or control of Jason Mitchell, or of other services.

The report was published by Gerald Duckworth & Co Ltd, The Old Piano Factory, 48 Hoxton Square, London N1 6PB (0171-729-5986) on 27th March 1996 - price £13.99.

REPORT OF AN INDEPENDENT JOINT AGENCY REVIEW FOR SOUTHAMPTON COMMUNITY HEALTH SERVICES NHS TRUST AND HAMPSHIRE COUNTY COUNCIL SOCIAL SERVICES DEPARTMENT INTO THE CIRCUMSTANCES SURROUNDING THE DEATHS OF GC, PJ AND TA

Dr Matt Muijen

GC, PJ and TA all died alone at home during the months of June and July 1995. Each of the three men was known to the Waterside and Romsey Community Mental Health Team, to the Department of Psychiatry, and to social services (either through social workers based in the team or, in one case, through the local Area Office). On 31st August 1995 the Southampton Coroner reached a open verdict on the cause of death of TA. On the 19th September a verdict of suicide was made in respect of PJ and an open verdict in the case of GC.

The published part of the review gives no details of the three men but an article headed "Starving man died while dog was cared for" appeared in the Daily Telegraph on 2nd September 1995:

"A man who gave away his dog because he could not afford to feed it was left to die in his council home. Tim Anstey was pale, thin and very weak when he contacted the RSPCA about his dog, Dusty. The cross-bred terrier was taken away at his request by a dog warden who reported Mr Anstey's condition to social services. Police also made reports but care workers failed to visit Mr Anstey at his home in Calmore, Southampton. His body was found by police more than two weeks later, an inquest was told. At the time of his death, Mr Anstey, 44, who lived alone and was not married was under a supervision order after being convicted of assaulting two police officers in June 1994. But probation officers had not visited him since April 12th - three months before he was found dead - when they warned him that he was in breach of his obligations by failing to attend probation appointments. Social services, the probation service and Southampton Community Health Services Trust are now conducting an inquiry into his death. After they discovered his body on July 20, police found a calendar marked with 50 consecutive days in which he had not eaten, and a series of unpaid bills for electricity, rent and court fines totalling nearly £1,000. ..."

The joint agency review, dated January 1996, was reported to the Trust Board and to the Adult Services Sub-Committee of the Hampshire County Council Social Services Committee.

1995

THE GREY REPORT: REPORT OF THE INDEPENDENT INQUIRY TEAM INTO THE CARE AND TREATMENT OF KENNETH GREY

Jane Mishcon, Dr Donald Dick, Nicholas Welch, Antony Sheehan, and Jane Mackay

Kenneth Grey was born in 1970. From the age of about 13, he started to use cannabis and then began to steal in order to buy drugs. The majority of his convictions were for burglary and theft and he had also been convicted for possessing cannabis on a number of occasions. He had three convictions for offences of violence. In June 1994, Kenneth Grey appeared in court charged with shoplifting (one whilst on bail for earlier offences) and one charge of common assault which arose from an assault on a store detective whom he hit because he would not release him when he was apprehended. Prior to sentencing, he was the subject of extensive probation assessments which indicated that he had a serious drug problem. It was acknowledged by the probation officers that he could not address his offending behaviour without first dealing with his drug problem, and one of the proposals in the reports was that he should be remanded on bail while an assessment was made at Phoenix House, a residential drug rehabilitation centre. He was accepted by Phoenix House following an assessment and funding was agreed. However, he absconded after only one day. He was sentenced to 12 months imprisonment and sent to Pentonville Prison.

While in custody, his behaviour began to be more and more bizarre until in October 1994, he was seen by one of the medical officers at Pentonville Prison. By this time he was expressing grandiose and delusional ideas and was seen in mid-October 1994 by a locum consultant psychiatrist from the Psychiatric Intensive Care Unit at Hackney Hospital, who did not consider him as being mentally ill at that time. Kenneth Grey had no prior history of any mental illness. His health deteriorated and by mid-November he had become threatening towards staff and other patients, and was displaying increasingly bizarre and grandiose ideas. He was seen at Pentonville by a forensic psychiatrist who carried out an assessment and considered him to be floridly mentally ill and he was transferred to the Psychiatric Intensive Care Unit (PICU) of Hackney Hospital on the 23rd November 1994 under s.47 of the Mental Health Act 1983. However, the s.47 Order was replaced two days later by a s.2 MHA Order, under the mistaken belief that the s.47 expired on Kenneth Grey's earliest date of release with remission (ie. 25th November 1994).

In the afternoon of the 2nd December 1994, the s.2 Order was discharged almost immediately prior to his transfer from the secure ward to an open ward. Within 2 hours of arriving on the open ward, he went missing from the Hospital and never returned.

On the evening of the 1st January 1995, Kenneth Grey killed his mother, apparently following an argument with her about religion. He was arrested immediately and it is clear that he was psychotic at the time of the homicide. He was charged with the murder of his mother and on the 25th July 1995 he appeared at the Old Bailey where his guilty plea to manslaughter on the grounds of diminished responsibility was accepted. Expert psychiatric evidence was called by both the prosecution and the defence, but the sentencing Judge was apparently persuaded by the evidence of the prosecution expert that Kenneth Grey was suffering from a drug induced psychosis at the time of the murder and that he was no longer showing any signs of mental illness.

Kenneth Grey was sentenced to 7 years imprisonment, but the Attorney General's authority has been obtained to refer Kenneth Grey's sentence to the Court of Appeal on the basis that it is unduly lenient.

The terms of reference of the Inquiry were to:

- investigate all of the circumstances prior to, and surrounding the admission, treatment and continuing care of Kenneth Grey - his leaving hospital and the death of his mother;
- examine the extent to which his care corresponded to statutory and other obligations of the Mental Health Act 1983 and all the relevant guidance from the Department of Health;
- identify any deficiencies in the quality and delivery of that care, both the internal and external collaboration and individual agency responsibilities;
- examine the effectiveness of the practice and the exercise of individual agency responsibilities in respect of absence without leave;
- make recommendations for the future assessment and care of people in similar circumstances including the mentally disordered so as to avoid possible harm to parents and the public;
- prepare the report including the recommendations to East London and the City Health Authority.

The report was published in November 1995 by East London & The City Health Authority, Tredegar House, 97-99 Bow Road, London E3 2AN (0181-983-2900) - price £10.

REPORT OF THE ENQUIRY INTO THE CARE AND TREATMENT OF PHILIP McFADDEN

Dr James Dyer, Dr Elizabeth McCall-Smith, John Sutherland, Jamie Malcolm

Philip McFadden was born in 1975. He began to show signs of mental illness in 1990 and was, for 8 months, a patient in the adolescent unit of Gartnavel Royal Hospital. He continued to have medication and psychiatric contact for the next two years. He was living with his family and his mother contacted the GP practice on several times on 17th June concerned about his mental state. The police went to the home which resulted in the death of a 28 year old police constable, Lewis Fulton, and a knife wound to another policeman. Philip McFadden was to have been tried on charges including murder and attempted murder but, at the High Court in Edinburgh in September 1994, was found insane in bar of trial and was sent to the State Hospital at Carstairs under s.174 of the Criminal Procedure (Scotland) Act 1975.

On 27th October 1994 the Secretary of State for Scotland wrote to the Chairman of the Mental Welfare Commission for Scotland asking the Commission to make enquiry under the duty placed upon it by s.3(2)(e), Mental Health (Scotland) Act 1984. As Philip McFadden had been found insane in bar of trial, it is possible that a trial might take place in the future should he recover to the necessary extent. It was therefore important that the Commission's enquiry should avoid any possibility of prejudice to a future trial, and that it should concern itself only with the psychiatric care and treatment received by Philip McFadden and not with the circumstances of the incident involving the police.

The terms of reference of the Inquiry, set up in November 1994, were to:

- examine the care and treatment received or not received by Philip McFadden, both in relation to the time around the incident of 17th June 1994 and also during an earlier period of mental illness which began in 1990.

The report was published by the Scottish Office, Department of Health, Room 29D, St Andrew's House, Edinburgh EH1 3DG.

THE BRIAN DOHERTY INQUIRY: REPORT OF THE INQUIRY TEAM TO THE WESTERN HEALTH AND SOCIAL SERVICES BOARD

Professor George Fenton, Eamonn Deane, Stanley Herron and Brendan Mullen

Brian Doherty was born in 1974. At the age of 6 he was assessed as "borderline educationally subnormal". He had contact, with twenty different caring agencies over a ten year period prior to the killing. These included special schools, children's homes, a training school, various young offender institutions, the Probation Service, and various hospitals. There was no evidence of a formal mental illness but a diagnosis of severe personality disorder of the dissocial type and mild mental handicap. This dual diagnosis caused placement problems.

He had a number of admissions to various hospitals as both a formal and informal patient. He was admitted to Tyrone and Fermanagh Hospital on 13th January 1994 (his second informal admission that month) following referral from the Accident and Emergency Department of Tyrone County

Hospital. He discharged himself, contrary to medical advice at 5pm on the 18th January 1994. Later that day he abducted and killed Kieran Hegarty, aged 11. On 15th May 1995, he pleaded guilty to manslaughter on the grounds of diminished responsibility and kidnapping and was sentenced to life imprisonment for manslaughter and ten years for kidnapping.

The terms of reference of the Inquiry were to:

- review and examine the circumstances surrounding the admission and discharge of Brian Doherty to and from the Tyrone and Fermanagh Hospital with particular reference to the applicability of the provisions of the Mental Health (Northern Ireland) Order 1986;

- make recommendations on operational policy and related changes in management arrangements arising from the experience learned from this incident. Such recommendations should also include any identified action;

- prepare a report of any relevant findings or recommendations arising out of this review for the Western Health and Social Services Board and the Mental Health Commission. The Western Health and Social Services Board will report its conclusions to the Minister for Health.

The report was published in October 1995 by the Western Health and Social Services Board, 15 Gransha Park, Clooney Rd, Londonderry, Northern Ireland BT47 1TG (01504-860086).

THE WOODLEY TEAM REPORT: REPORT OF THE INDEPENDENT REVIEW PANEL TO EAST LONDON AND THE CITY HEALTH AUTHORITY AND NEWHAM COUNCIL

Len Woodley QC, Ken Dixon, Vivien Lindow, Dr Oyedeji Oyebode, Tom Sandford and Stephen Simblet

Stephen Laudat was born in 1968. His mother suffered from mental illness. In 1991 he was jailed for 4 years in 1991 for thefts and robberies, one involving a knife. His mental health deteriorated in prison and he was transferred under ss.47/49, Mental Health Act 1983 initially to the Interim Secure Unit at Hackney Hospital and, in June 1992, to Kneesworth House Hospital. He was discharged from Kneesworth House on his earliest release date in December 1993. In July 1994 he stabbed to death Bryan Bennett, aged 56, at a Day Centre in Newham where both attended. In December 1994, Stephen Laudat was sent to Rampton Hospital under ss.37/41 after he admitted manslaughter on the grounds of diminished responsibility.

The terms of reference of the Inquiry were to:

- investigate all circumstances surrounding the incident;

- take due regard of all previous and on-going assessment, treatment and care, both planned for or received by Stephen Laudat;

- evaluate the extent to which the care and treatment corresponded with statutory obligations, relevant guidance from the Department of Health and local operational policies and procedures;

- assess the quality, range and delivery of the care and treatment, including assessments of risk, and whether it was suitable for his needs;

- evaluate the adequacy of arrangements for inter-agency collaboration, their effectiveness in practice and the exercise of individual responsibilities;
- make recommendations for the future delivery, quality and range of care and treatment available to mentally ill people, including the safety of mental health users, the public and staff.
- prepare a report and make recommendations to East London and The City Health Authority and Newham Social Services Committee; to summarise its main findings for distribution to other interested parties.

The commissioning authorities drew attention to a number of more detailed points relating to the above terms of reference, as background information.

- Stephen Laudat's social history, childhood experience, contact with criminal justice agencies and, particularly, the treatment and care provided for him since 1989;
- The likely influence of any assumptions about his race and background on his social, housing, medical and psychiatric care;
- Existing reports which are relevant to Newham's mental health services, including from the Mental Health Act Commission, the Mental Health Task Force, the Social Services Inspection and Quality Assurance Unit, plus Public Health reports and reports on Newham's needs;
- The history and effectiveness of any medication regime, bearing in mind his psychiatric diagnosis and his response to treatment;
- Any health and safety issues which are pertinent to the range of services provided at the Worland Centre and the diversity of service users;
- The specific needs of Newham's population, with particular reference to the resourcing of mental health services and its impact on this case;
- The Care Programme Approach.

The report was published in September 1995 by East London and The City Health Authority, Tredegar House, 97-99 Bow Rd, London E3 2AN (0181-983-2900) - price £10.

REPORT OF THE INQUIRY INTO THE CIRCUMSTANCES LEADING TO THE DEATH OF JONATHAN NEWBY (A VOLUNTEER WORKER)

Nicola Davies QC, Richard Lingham, Clifford Prior, Professor Andrew Sims

John Rous was born in 1946. He was first admitted to a psychiatric hospital in 1965 for an amphetamine psychosis, when a diagnosis of personality disorder was made. He had several further admissions under the provisions of the Mental Health Act 1959. He had a street life of some twenty years before he took up residence in Jacqui Porter House, run by Oxford Cyrenians, in August 1992. Jonathan Newby began working for the Cyrenians as a volunteer in April 1993 and was the only person on duty when he was attacked by John Rous in the office of Jacqui Porter House. He was 22 years old when he died. John Rous subsequently admitted manslaughter on the grounds of diminished responsibility and was sent to Broadmoor Hospital under ss.37/41, Mental Health Act 1983.

The terms of reference of the Inquiry, set up in July 1994, were to:

- examine all the circumstances surrounding the treatment and continuing care of John Rous, in particular:

  The appropriateness of the care plan and care provided in the context of John Rous's history and his assessed health and social care needs;

  The extent to which John Rous's care corresponded to statutory obligations, relevant guidance from the Department of Health, discharge guidance and local operational policies;

  The history of John Rous's prescribed medication and compliance with that medication.

- examine the circumstances regarding the admission of John Rous's to Jacqui Porter House including:

  The suitability of the placement in view of his history and assessed health and social care needs;

  To comment upon the organisation of the hostel and the quality of care provided in Jacqui Porter House at the time of Jonathan Newby's death;

- examine the adequacy of the arrangements for collaboration and communication between the agencies (Oxfordshire Mental Health Unit - now the Oxfordshire Mental Healthcare NHS Trust, Oxfordshire SSD, the Elmore Community Support Team, Oxford City Council Housing Department, Oxford Cyrenians) involved in the care of John Rous;

- prepare a report and make recommendations to the Chairman, Oxfordshire Health Authority.

The report was published in July 1995 by Oxfordshire Health, Old Rd, Headington, Oxford OX3 7LF (01865-741741) - price £10.

REPORT OF THE INDEPENDENT PANEL OF INQUIRY INTO THE CIRCUMSTANCES SURROUNDING THE DEATHS OF ELLEN AND ALAN BOLAND

Mrs J Hughes, Mrs L Mason, Dr R Pinto and Mr P Williams

Alan Boland suffered from depression and alcoholism. He was, over a period of nine years, seen by over 20 doctors whilst an outpatient at the Paterson Wing. He commenced attending the Day Hospital in November 1993. On the evening of 5th March 1994, it is alleged that he came home to the flat which he shared with his mother, aged 71, strangled her and hit her repeatedly about the head with a hammer. He spent the rest of the night in the flat, though upstairs in his own bedroom, leaving around midday on 6th March by the fire escape which meant he did not have to pass his mother's body in the hall. He spent the rest of that day drinking. He returned to the flat at about **11pm** where he was arrested. On 25th July 1994, whilst on remand, he was found dead in his cell at Wandsworth Prison, having hanged himself.

The terms of reference of the Inquiry were to:

- establish the history of contacts by Alan Boland and his mother with statutory or other agencies, including the North West London Mental Health NHS Trust and the Housing and Social Services Departments of the City of Westminster, until his death;

- assess whether the actions of, and the liaison within and between, the agencies involved were adequate and appropriate;

- assess whether it was appropriate for Alan Boland to have been discharged from hospital care at the Paterson Wing in February 1994, to identify the arrangements that were made for his continuing care, and to assess whether those arrangements were appropriate to his needs;

- establish whether any of the agencies involved had any reason to anticipate that he might have been a danger to his mother or to himself, and, if so, whether all appropriate and reasonable steps were taken to notify other agencies, and, by them, to act upon such;

- present to the commissioning agencies a report, including conclusions and recommendations, which will be made public.

The report was published in March 1995 by the North West London Mental Health NHS Trust, IKEA Tower, 255 North Circular Road, Brent Park, London NW10 0JQ (0181-830-0033).

THE FALLING SHADOW: ONE PATIENT'S MENTAL HEALTH CARE 1978 - 1993

Sir Louis Blom-Cooper QC, Helen Hally and Professor Elaine Murphy

Andrew Robinson was born in 1957. He was first admitted to a psychiatric unit in 1977. In 1978, following conviction for carrying a firearm with intent to endanger the life of a female university student, and assault occasioning actual bodily harm, he was made the subject of a Hospital Order with restrictions and admitted to Broadmoor Hospital. He was transferred to a local hospital in 1981 and conditionally discharged in 1983. Andrew Robinson was admitted on seven occasions to the Edith Morgan Centre between 1986 and his last admission on 9th June 1993 when he was initially detained as an emergency (s.4, Mental Health Act 1983) and then the following day reassessed and detained for treatment.

On 1st September 1993, Georgina Robinson, aged 27, an occupational therapist at the Edith Morgan Centre at Torbay District Hospital was fatally wounded by Andrew Robinson who was still detained under s.3, Mental Health Act 1983. Georgina Robinson subsequently died on 7th October 1993. Andrew Robinson pleaded guilty to manslaughter on the grounds of diminished responsibility and was detained under a hospital order with restrictions (ss.37/41, Mental Health Act 1983) and readmitted to Broadmoor Hospital.

The terms of reference of the Inquiry, set up in September 1993, were to:

- investigate what actually happened on 1st September 1993 at the Edith Morgan Centre;
- investigate Andrew Robinson's clinical history, so far as known and relevant to matters under review; and his involvement with mental health services, in particular, services in the Torbay area during the period leading up to his admission to the Edith Morgan Centre;
- consider the lessons and implications arising, with a view to making recommendations. This is likely to include consideration of the following matters:

  the influences of architectural factors, and the possible modification to the Edith Morgan Centre itself, and to the client group admitted and treated there;

  the state of the art of the assessment of risk and prediction of dangerousness posed by patients;

  the control and discipline of psychiatric patients - in particular, how incidents caused by patients are managed by staff;

  the availability of hospital beds in other facilities, such as the Butler Clinic, the special hospital system, so far as this affects the sound management of the Edith Morgan Centre.

The Inquiry also took evidence about the circumstances of the death of Stephen Hext, aged 21, who fell from the roof of a multi-storey car park. At that time he was on leave from the Edith Morgan Centre where he was an informal patient.

The report was published in January 1995 by Gerald Duckworth & Co Ltd, The Old Piano Factory, 48 Hoxton Square, London N1 6PB (0171-729-5986) - price £12.99.

1994

INQUIRY INTO THE DEATHS OF JASON AND NATALIA HARRY

Jean Gabbott and Dr Oscar Hill

Sharon Dalson was born in 1969. Her two children Jason and Natalia Harry were placed on the Child Protection Register in 1988 after they were left on their own but removed from the Register in June 1991. In December 1991, she was taken to hospital by the Police under s.136, Mental Health Act 1983 and subsequently detained under s.2, Mental Health Act 1983. She was discharged a week later but arrested later that month after she held a knife to the children's throats and threatened suicide. In February 1992 she was detained in hospital under s.37, Mental Health Act 1983. In April 1992 she was given "trial leave" and returned home and began attending the Day Hospital. Her children, who were being cared for by their grandmother, were placed on the Child Protection Register in June 1992.

In August 1992 Sharon Dalson strangled Jason, aged six and suffocated Natalia, aged five. She admitted the manslaughter of her children and was sent to Rampton Hospital.

The terms of reference of the Inquiry, set up in September 1992, were to:

- receive the Management review reports and recommendations of each agency involved including actions already taken;
- consider the actions taken by agencies within the relevant guidance e.g. Working Together, Haringey Council and Health Department and Police guidelines and to enquire into any matters in relation to agency actions.
- report to Haringey Area Child Protection Committee on the findings of the Inquiry and the recommendations for future action that agencies may wish to take and that such findings be made public subsequent to the conclusion of any criminal or coroner investigation which may be undertaken.

The report was completed in September 1994 and a summary is available from Haringey Child Protection Committee, 3rd Floor, Duke House, Crouch End, London N8 8HE.

REPORT OF THE INDEPENDENT PANEL OF INQUIRY EXAMINING THE CASE OF MICHAEL BUCHANAN

Christopher Heginbotham, Jacqueline Carr, Dr Robert Hale, Thomas Walsh and Linda Warren

Michael Buchanan was born on 31st July 1964. He was first admitted to a psychiatric hospital in 1983 and was subsequently admitted on a further 12 occasions. He was last admitted on 31st July 1992 to Shenley Hospital under s.37, Mental Health Act 1983. Following a s.117 Mental Health Act 1983 aftercare meeting on 18th August 1992 he was discharged on 21st August 1992 after 22 days on the ward to a Church Army Hostel. On 10th September 1992, Michael Buchanan entered an underground car park on the Stonebridge Park Estate, Harlesden. In the car park Frederick Graver, a 54 year old former policeman, had just parked his car. Michael Buchanan picked up a piece of wood and attacked him, knocking him to the ground. He hit Frederick Graver about the head with the wood and stamped on his face with great force causing 13 severe multiple fractures to his facial bones and he died two days later.

The terms of reference of the Inquiry, set up in October 1993, were to:

- examine the circumstances leading to, and the arrangements for, Michael Buchanan's admission to Shenley Hospital;
- examine the adequacy of the treatment and patient management including the discharge planning for Michael Buchanan from Shenley Hospital;
- examine the concepts of mental disorder applied in this case and the implications for treatment;
- examine the post discharge care and all the after care arrangements for Michael Buchanan, provided by North West London Trust and other agencies;
- consider whether a wider review of the public policy context within which this case is situated should be undertaken;

- consider the treatment and care for patients with similar combinations of disorders;
- prepare a report and recommendations to the North West London Mental Health NHS Trust.

The report was published in November 1994 by the North West London Mental Health NHS Trust, IKEA Tower, 255 North Circular Road, Brent Park, London NW10 0JQ (0181-830-0033).

REPORT OF THE INQUIRY INTO ASPECTS OF LEARNING DISABILITIES SERVICES MANAGED BY THAMESIDE COMMUNITY HEALTHCARE NHS TRUST

Norman Warner, Heather Rendle and Tom Freeman

This followed concerns raised by relatives and the local Community Health Council in respect of 6 patients with learning difficulties. Complaints included issues surrounding the investigation of complaints and communications with relatives.

The terms of reference of the Inquiry, set up in January 1994, were to:

- review complaints (and the resulting inquiries since 1991 investigating the standards of care provided at South Ockendon Hospital and within staffed community homes) and report whether the recommendations of those investigations were acted upon correctly;
- identify whether policies and procedures recently introduced, including complaints procedures, are adequate for the future and suitable for community care;
- make recommendations as appropriate.

The report was published in May 1994 by Thameside Community Healthcare NHS Trust, Thurrock Community Hospital, Long Lane, Grays, Essex RM16 2PX (01375-390044).

SOUTH DEVON HEALTHCARE TRUST

Sir Louis Blom-Cooper QC, Helen Hally and Professor Elaine Murphy

A cluster of 10 suicides of patients, or recent former patients, of the service between June 1988 and June 1989 caused local concern about the style of service and about the management of the Edith Morgan Unit. Various review reports over the preceding 7 years had commented on:

- the fragmentation and lack of co-ordination between the inpatient and community based parts of the service;
- the serious lack of professional leadership, especially in the inpatient services;
- the unsuitability of the Edith Morgan Centre for acute psychiatric inpatient work in terms of its siting, lay-out, size and integration with community services;

- the inability of the services to manage seriously disturbed people with difficult behaviours and the lack of appropriate facilities for this group.

The terms of reference of the Inquiry, set up in October 1993, were to:

- study and report on the mental health care in South Devon, with special references to the general acute services; and to make recommendations.

The report was published in April 1994 by South Devon Healthcare Trust, Torbay Hospital, Lawes Bridge, Torquay, Devon TQ2 7AA (01803-614567).

REPORT OF THE INQUIRY INTO THE CARE AND TREATMENT OF CHRISTOPHER CLUNIS

Jean Ritchie QC, Dr Donald Dick and Richard Lingham

Christopher Clunis was born in 1963. Both his parents came from Jamaica. He began to show odd behaviour in 1986 and went to stay with his father in Jamaica. He was subsequently admitted to Bellevue Hospital, Kingston, Jamaica where he was diagnosed as having paranoid schizophrenia. He returned to London the following year and was admitted to various psychiatric hospitals on a number of occasions in the following years. On 20th August 1992, Christopher Clunis was detained under s.3, Mental Health Act 1983 and transferred the following day from Kneesworth House to Guys Hospital. He was discharged on 24th September 1992 to accommodation in Haringey. On 17th December 1992, Christopher Clunis stabbed Jonathan Zito, a complete stranger, to death in an unprovoked attack at Finsbury Park Tube Station. On the day of the murder an Approved Social Worker visited Christopher Clunis' address unaccompanied, leaving a note asking him to call and see her. He was by then in custody. He pleaded guilty to manslaughter at the Old Bailey on 28th June 1993 and sent to Rampton Hospital under ss.37/41, Mental Health Act 1983.

The terms of reference of the Inquiry, set up in July 1993, were to:

- investigate all the circumstances surrounding the admission, treatment, discharge and continuing care of Christopher Clunis between May and December 1992;

- identify any deficiencies in the quality and delivery of that care, as well as inter-agency collaboration and individual responsibilities;

- make recommendations for the future delivery of care including admission, treatment, discharge and continuing care to people in similar circumstances so that, as far as possible, harm to patients and the public is avoided.

The report was published in February 1994 by HMSO - price £9.50.

An examination of the information compiled by the Inquiry Team and an analysis of the validity of their conclusions from the perspective of Race Equality by Vernon Harris entitled *A Review of the Report of the Inquiry into the Care and Treatment of Christopher Clunis - A black perspective* is published by the Race Equality Unit, 5 Tavistock Place, London WC1H 9SN - price £7.

NORTH WEST LONDON MENTAL HEALTH SERVICES INQUIRY

Margaret Goose, Catherine McLoughlin and Dr David Owens

The inquiry arose from the concerns of the General Manager of the then Parkside Health Authority that there appeared to have been an unduly high number of 'serious incidents' within the Mental Health Unit, Parkside District. Of the 21 incidents examined, 10 of these involved deaths which were definite or probable suicides and 4 were episodes of non-fatal self harm. There were 4 deaths of patients from a physical illness, 2 cases involved alleged sexual assault by one patient on another and the final case involved attacks on staff.

The terms of reference of the Inquiry, set up in March 1993, were to:

- investigate all aspects relating to 21 untoward incidents involving 20 patients of the Unit between 1st March 1991 and 31st January 1993;
- consider any other current reports on issues in the Unit and whether these are pertinent to the investigation (e.g. reports of the Health Service Commissioner, Mental Health Act Commission, etc.);
- review the quality of the standards of medical and nursing care, supervision and monitoring of medical and nursing staff in training, multi-disciplinary working, organisation and management of services;
- review the management of these 21 untoward incidents, the action taken and the reporting arrangements;
- make recommendations in the light of the findings.

The report was published in February 1994 by the North West London Mental Health NHS Trust, IKEA Tower, 255 North Circular Road, Brent Park, London NW10 0JQ (0181-830-0033).

1993

REPORT OF THE INQUIRY PANEL TO INVESTIGATE THE SERIOUS UNTOWARD INCIDENT AT THE TUDOR REST HOME, NOTTINGHAM

Mrs. P. Turnbull, Dr. O. Oyebode, Mr J Archer

David Usoro was born in 1965. Between March 1990 and September 1992 he was admitted to Mapperley Hospital, Nottingham on seven occasions, including under s.3, Mental Health Act 1983. The clinical diagnosis was bipolar affective disorder - manic episode on each occasion. The diagnosis was complicated by a persistent history of solvent abuse. There was also evidence supporting the additional diagnosis of personality disorder. On 1st September 1992 he was discharged from Mapperley Hospital to live in his own flat. In April 1993 he moved into the Tudor Rest Home, registered to take seven residents, as he was not coping very well.

On 2nd August 1993 David Usoro was visited by a Senior Registrar in Psychiatry and a Community Psychiatric Nurse who found him to be excitable, over familiar and with pressure of speech. He would not agree to informal admission and assessed as not meeting the criteria for formal admission. The following evening, he attacked two residents with a knife, fatally wounding Samuel Vernon, aged 59. He was subsequently detained in a Special Hospital.

The terms of reference of the Panel were to:

- establish the facts and examine the actions of those concerned with the events, leading to the arrest of a resident, which took place at Tudor Rest Home, Nottingham from 1st to 4th August 1993;
- consider the management and treatment of the five residents of the residential home who were under the care and supervision of the Nottingham Healthcare Unit;
- make such recommendations to the District Health Authority as may be considered necessary in the light of the findings.

The Panel reported in November 1993 to Nottingham Health Authority, Forest House, Berkeley Avenue, Nottingham NG3 5AF.

REPORT OF THE COMMITTEE OF INQUIRY INTO THE DEATH IN BROADMOOR HOSPITAL OF ORVILLE BLACKWOOD AND A REVIEW OF THE DEATHS OF TWO OTHER AFRO-CARIBBEAN PATIENTS "BIG, BLACK, AND DANGEROUS?"

Professor Herschel Prins, Tony Backer-Holst, Errol Francis and Dr Ian Keitch

Orville Blackwood was born in Jamaica in 1960 and came to the UK at an early age with his mother. He came to psychiatric attention in 1982 and in the next 4 years was compulsorily admitted to psychiatric hospitals on 8 occasions (once through the Courts) before being convicted of robbery and possession of an imitation firearm (a toy gun at a bookmakers). In April 1986 he was sentenced to imprisonment of 3 years and 1 year respectively, sentences to run concurrently. He was transferred to HMP Grendon Underwood and then in January 1987 admitted to a Regional Secure Unit. He was transferred to Broadmoor in October 1987 under ss.47/49, Mental Health Act 1983. His Earliest Date of Release was September 1988. On the morning of 28th August 1991, Orville Blackwood went voluntarily into a seclusion room in Broadmoor Hospital and, when reviewed that afternoon, was restrained and injected with 150mg Sparine and 150mg Modecate. He died almost immediately. The pathologist gave the cause of death as "Cardiac failure associated with the administration of phenothiazine drugs".

The terms of reference of the Inquiry, set up in September 1991, were to:

- investigate the circumstances leading to the death of Orville Blackwood in Broadmoor Hospital on 28th August 1991;
- examine the reports of the inquiries into the deaths of Michael Martin and Joseph Watts in the same hospital to identify any significant common factors between all three deaths;
- make appropriate recommendations to the Special Hospitals Service Authority for future policies and actions.

The report was published by the Special Hospitals Service Authority in 1993 and is currently out of print.

1992

INDEPENDENT INQUIRY INTO THE CARE AND TREATMENT OF KEVIN ROONEY

Andrew Collins QC, Dr Oscar Hill and Michael Taylor

Kevin Rooney was born in 1963. He was first admitted in September 1985 under s.4, Mental Health Act 1983 to Claybury Hospital after he threatened his family with a pair of scissors and a hatchet. He was compulsorily readmitted to psychiatric hospitals on a number of occasions in the following years. Late at night on 3rd May 1991, Kevin Rooney was taken to the accident and emergency department of Homerton Hospital by the police after a woman had complained that he had threatened her in the lift of a block of flats with what she thought was a knife but was in fact a cooking spatula. He had a shirt tied round his head like a turban as he believed he was a Sikh and had delusions that he was being persecuted which he said was the reason he had threatened the woman in the lift. He was admitted informally at 1.30 am on 4th May 1991 but was found to be missing at 4.30pm the following day. On 7th May he was discharged in his absence following a discussion in the course of the routine ward round. On 9th May he visited his GP who was not available. The receptionist was scared as he holding a closed lock knife. He refused to see another doctor and said he would return the following day to see his own GP. He did not return and his GP informed the hospital who was told that he had left the hospital several days earlier and had been discharged in his absence. On 11th May 1991 Kevin Rooney stabbed Grace Quigley, whom he had known from the previous year when she had also been a patient at Hackney Hospital, 28 times with a lock knife in the presence of her children and a neighbour. He was arrested by police, who were called to the scene, since he remained waiting at a nearby bus stop. He was charged with murder and on 13th January 1992 at the Central Criminal Court he pleaded guilty to manslaughter on the grounds of diminished responsibility and sent to Rampton Hospital under ss.37/41, Mental Health Act 1983.

The terms of reference of the Inquiry, set up in April 1992 at the request of the Secretary of State for Health, were to:

- inquire into the arrangements for the assessment, care, discharge and follow up of Kevin Rooney by the mental health and related services in City and Hackney HA and North East Thames RHA;
- consider the adequacy of these arrangements;
- report their findings and to recommend any action which, in the light of these, might assist the assessment and care of mentally disabled patients and the protection of those patients and the public from the risk of harm.

The report was published in December 1992 by North Thames Regional Health Authority, 40 Eastbourne Terrace, London W2 3QR.

FINDINGS OF THE INDEPENDENT REVIEW ON THE MANAGEMENT OF THE CASE OF ERIEYUNE INWEH

Dr Gordon Langley and Rick Willis

Erieyune (Erhi) Inweh was born in 1970. She was first admitted to hospital in July 1991 and, after treatment whilst detained under s.3, Mental Health Act 1983, was discharged in October 1991 to a short-term aftercare hostel run by Kingston MIND. In August 1992 she was detained by police under s.136, Mental Health Act 1983 and taken to hospital where she was subsequently detained under s.2, Mental Health Act 1983. She was discharged and returned to the MIND hostel in September 1992.

On 30th October 1992, at approximately 9.20am, Catherine (Katie) Sullivan, aged 23, a voluntary worker at the MIND hostel was fatally stabbed 14 times. Erhi Inweh was subsequently detained in Broadmoor Hospital.

The terms of reference of this Independent Review were to:

- undertake an independent review of the management of the case of Erhi Inweh, from the time of her first admission to hospital in July 1991, to her arrest on a charge of the murder of Catherine Sullivan, on 30th October 1992.

- include an analysis of case records and interviews with key staff involved in working with Erhi Inweh, and to consider and report on the following:
  - The initial assessment and subsequent reviews undertaken;
  - The decisions reached in the case;
  - The care plans/treatment offered;
  - The appropriateness of the residential placement;
  - The nature and level of support given by all agencies concerned.

The Independent Review was completed in December 1992.

COMMITTEE OF INQUIRY INTO THE DEATH OF FREDA LATHAM AT STALLINGTON HOSPITAL

Tony Bell, David Caswell, Dr Myrtle Summerly, Wendy Thornley and Paul Bishop

Freda Latham, aged 43, a long-standing patient in Stallington Hospital, was taken to the toilet area by a staff nurse at approximately 1pm on 13th May 1992. After she was washed she was taken to a toilet cubicle and seated on the toilet and the tapes of her bib were secured to the inlet pipe of the toilet cistern. After she was tied to the pipe she was left unattended and the staff nurse went to lunch. The Acting Charge Nurse later entered the cubicle and gave her medication before also going to lunch and leaving Freda Latham in the toilet. At approximately 1.45pm, a member of the domestic staff discovered Freda Latham in the toilet and she was certified dead at 2.10pm. The cause of death was inhalation of vomit and suspension.

The terms of reference of the Inquiry were to:

- examine the circumstances leading up to the death of Freda Latham;
- examine the levels of staffing and supervision of those staff on Erica Ward;
- assess the experience and skill mix of the staff on duty at the time of the death;
- assess the effectiveness and level of control exerted by nurse management;
- look at the care and attention of the acutely mentally handicapped residents on Erica Ward.

The report was published by N. Staffordshire Health Authority in October 1992.

REPORT OF THE COMMITTEE OF INQUIRY INTO COMPLAINTS ABOUT ASHWORTH HOSPITAL

Sir Louis Blom-Cooper QC, Martin Brown, Dr Robert Dolan and Professor Elaine Murphy

The terms of reference of the inquiry, set up in April 1991, were to:

- investigate allegations of improper care and treatment at Ashworth Hospital contained within the "Cutting Edge" documentary *A Special Hospital* transmitted on 4th May 1991, and any other relevant allegations brought to their attention;

- in the light of these investigations, to review the arrangements for handling complaints by or on behalf of patients about the care or treatment provided at Ashworth Hospital, including arrangements for the reference of complaints (where appropriate) to the relevant police force, and to report their findings and to make recommendations for action in respect of these matters.

In September 1991 the Inquiry was put on a statutory footing (s.125, Mental Health Act 1983) and the terms of reference were minimally amended to take into account the fact that some evidence had already been taken.

The inquiry looked at 10 cases for the purpose of examining the application of hospital's complaints system and hospital management's actions in response. A further four cases were singled out for in-depth examination:

- Sean Walton was committed to Moss Side Hospital in 1983 under ss.60/65, Mental Health Act 1959 on the grounds of subnormality within the meaning of the Act 1959 following an indecent assault on a four year old girl. He died suddenly at the age of 20 after sixteen hours in seclusion at Ashworth Hospital (formerly Moss Side and Park Lane Hospitals) on 1st March 1988;

- Geoffrey Steele was transferred to Ashworth Hospital in April 1990 from Reaside Regional Secure Unit and alleged that he had been physically assaulted by staff in the month following admission;

- Gillian Darnell had been a patient at the hospital since 1982 and alleged she had been sexually abused by a male nurse in 1985;

- Gary Harrington was transferred to Park Lane Hospital from Winson Green Prison under s.48, Mental Health Act 1983 in June 1987. While on remand in prison he made a number of attempts to self-harm, including a serious suicide attempt. He was recognised as a suicide risk on admission to Park Lane and within 3 months of admission he had "tested his door (wardrobe) for its weight - bearing capacity". Two other patients took their own life at the hospital in a similar way over the next couple of years before Gary Harrington hanged himself from the wardrobe door on 1st May 1990.

The report, presented to Parliament in August 1992, is published in two parts by HMSO. Volume I - price £26.60, and Volume II (case studies) - price £14.90.

The SHSA subsequently requested the Health Advisory Service to look at the Hospital two years on from the Inquiry, and to assess current strategy and achievements in the interval, as well as offer advice relating to any of the issues in the terms of reference. Their report "With care in mind secure" was published in March 1995 by the Health Advisory Service, 3rd Floor, Sutherland House, 29-37 Brighton Rd, Sutton, Surrey SM2 5AN (0181-642-6421).

REVIEW OF DEATHS AMONG PATIENTS OF OXFORDSHIRE HEALTH AUTHORITY MENTAL HEALTH UNIT: 1990 - 1991

Vivyenne Rubenstein

This inquiry followed an internal review carried out with the assistance of Professor Morgan, Department of Mental Health, University of Bristol. It examined the circumstances surrounding the death of 7 patients of the Mental Health Unit between July 1990 and July 1991. These were described in the report as:

- "Case A: Admitted as emergency GP referral voluntary patient. Treated for severe depression and suicidal thoughts. Took own life 13 days later while on leave from ward."

- "Case B: History of severe relapsing paranoid schizophrenia with multiple admissions. Experienced medication as torture and pain. Hostile towards staff. Unwilling to co-operate with close follow up regime. Recognised as suicide risk. Finally admitted under s.3 and after two months went on leave to own flat. Took own life 3 weeks later."

- "Case C: History of manic depressive psychosis with suicidal inclinations. Multiple admissions over the years, lately as out-patient. Transferred to in-patient care on a different ward following concerns about increased suicidal inclination. Discharged after 9 days to own flat as "observations did not support diagnosis of depressive illness". Failed to take up aftercare options. Died 2 weeks later. Open verdict."

- "Case D: History of schizo-affective psychosis. Multiple admissions. Initially very resistant to psychiatric help. Then admitted as voluntary patient seeking help in the face of greater recognition of his own plight. Viewed as high suicide risk. Died 4 weeks later while off hospital premises. Open verdict."

- "Case E: Suffered from Hebephrenic Schizophrenia, a particularly severe form resistant to medication. After 7 months in secure unit he was transferred to an open ward as a sectioned patient for a rehabilitation trial. Particular emphasis was placed on the need for urgent action should he abscond. Not thought to be a high suicide risk although family expressed concern over his depressed state in last days. Absconded and died on second day. Open verdict."

- "Case F: Severe relapsing schizophrenia. Multiple previous admissions, some under section. Opposed to medication. Attributed symptoms to medication rather than to the illness. Re-admitted after failed discharge to own flat. Perceived relationships with some staff as bad and felt insecure on ward. Family considered there was lack of recognition of his needs and the help they could give. Plans had been made for a progressive discharge back to the flat, Took own life on ward."

- "Case G: History of mental illness. Diagnosis initially schizophrenia, then chronic manic-depressive hypomania. Multiple admissions over a number of years. Opposed to some of the medication. Viewed symptoms as effect of drugs more than of the disease. Finally readmitted as voluntary patient when felt resurgence of manic phase. Some uninhibited behaviour. Perception by family of hostility and lack of insight from some staff. Disputed discharge after 1 month while still on high medication. Initiative for contact left to patient. Found dead 11 days later. Open verdict."

The report was published in March 1992 by Oxfordshire Health Authority, Manor House, Headley Way, Headington, Oxford OX3 9DZ.

REPORT OF THE INVESTIGATION INTO SERIOUS INCIDENTS OCCURRING AT THE SHRODELLS PSYCHIATRIC UNIT: OCTOBER 1989 - NOVEMBER 1990

This investigation followed an earlier inquiry in 1991 which was set up following the death of Margaret Price, aged 67, in December 1990 following an assault by a fellow patient. This inquiry revealed that in the 15 months prior to December 1990, a further 9 serious incidents had taken place. These were:-

- the death of a male patient aged 61 from an aspirin overdose,
- the treatment of a female patient aged 23 with anorexia who developed neuroleptic malignant syndrome,
- the arrest by police at the hospital of a male patient aged 28 who objected to being discharged,
- the absconding and death of a male patient aged 54 who had been assessed as a high suicide risk,
- the death from untreated hypertension of a female patient aged 42 with manic depression,
- self-injury by a depressed female patient aged 64 whilst under close observation,
- death from endocarditis of a male patient aged 46 with a cardiac pacemaker who was suffering from a paranoid illness,
- death of a male patient aged 39 with epilepsy and encephalitis who died while taking an unsupervised bath,
- death of a male patient aged 25 who absconded from hospital the day after admission and jumped from a bridge.

The terms of reference of the Inquiry, set up in 1991, were to:

- undertake a review of these 9 further incidents with a view to strengthening the mental health service in S.W. Hertfordshire for the safety and welfare of mentally ill patients.

The report was published in January 1992 by the S.W. Hertfordshire DHA.

1991

REPORT OF THE PANEL OF INQUIRY APPOINTED BY THE WEST MIDLANDS REGIONAL HEALTH AUTHORITY, SOUTH BIRMINGHAM HEALTH AUTHORITY AND THE SPECIAL HOSPITALS SERVICE AUTHORITY TO INVESTIGATE THE CASE OF KIM KIRKMAN

Dr Donald Dick, Barry Shuttleworth and John Charlton

Kim Kirkman was born in 1955. He was detained under ss.60/65, Mental Health Act 1959 following an assault whilst in hospital and admitted to Broadmoor Hospital in March 1973. He was transferred to Park Lane Hospital in 1983 and to the Reaside Regional Secure Unit in January 1989. In February 1990, the Home Secretary agreed to a conditional discharge and Kim Kirkman and his fiancee were helped to make an application for accommodation. The tenancy of a flat was offered and accepted. On 1st June 1990 he went to the flat for the day and returned to Reaside that evening. Later that day the body of Elizabeth Ford was found in her flat in the same house. Kim Kirkman was arrested and subsequently confessed. He was remanded to Winson Green Prison where he hung himself in his cell on 5th September 1990.

The terms of reference of the Inquiry were to:

- inquire into and report upon the diagnoses, management and treatment of Kim Kirkman, including the reasons for and surrounding his transfers from both Broadmoor and Ashworth Hospitals, and the reasons for and surrounding the arrangements for his discharge from in-patient care at the Reaside Clinic, Rubery, and his remand in custody to Winson Green Prison;

- consider the arrangements made, and the reasons for the discharge from in-patient care of patients who are subject to Court Orders under the Mental Health Act 1983, and to report, including reference to their use and operation, in respect of Kim Kirkman.

The report was published in November 1991 by the West Midlands RHA.

REGIONAL FACT FINDING COMMITTEE OF ENQUIRY INTO THE ADMISSION, CARE, TREATMENT AND DISCHARGE OF CAROL BARRATT

Cyril Unwin MBE, Dr D Morgan and B Smith

Carol Barratt was admitted under s.2, Mental Health Act 1983 to the Psychiatric Unit at Doncaster Royal Infirmary in March 1991 after threatening a young woman with a knife. On 4th April she absconded from the hospital and attacked a girl outside the hospital. On her return she attempted to strangle a visitor to the hospital. On 11th April she unsuccessfully appealed to a Mental Health Review Tribunal. On 14th April, Carol Barratt, who was on very close nursing observation, was visited by her mother who complained about some bruising on her arms. She actively encouraged her daughter to leave the ward and demanded she be discharged. Dr Silvester, the Responsible Medical Officer, allowed Carol Barratt to leave "against medical advice" after her mother gave an undertaking that she would take full responsibility for her. On 16th April 1991, Carol Barratt visited the Frenchgate Centre Shopping Precinct where she stabbed Emma Brodie, aged 11, in the chest and who subsequently died.

The terms of reference of the Inquiry, set up in May 1991, were to:

- examine the facts surrounding Carol Barratt's discharge from the Psychiatric Unit at Doncaster Royal Infirmary on 14th April 1991, and the relevant facts relating to her admission, care and treatment and to make recommendations in the light of its findings.

A summary of the Committee's conclusions and recommendations were published by Trent RHA in October 1991.

INQUIRY INTO THE NHS CARE, TREATMENT AND MANAGEMENT OF STEPHEN FINDLEY

Hugh FitzGerald, Colin Gatiss, Arthur Holroyd, Jane Johnston, Dr Marion Swan and Trevor Thompson.

Stephen Findley was born in 1968. He was admitted to hospital under s.2, Mental Health Act 1983 in November 1990 after being arrested by police following an incident at a night club where he was found to have in his possession a loaded Webley air pistol and two knives. It was decided that there were no grounds to detain him beyond the expiry of the s.2 order. He took his discharge, against medical advice the following day. Five days later he attacked Oliver Dickens, aged 67, a passer-by in the street, stabbing him 32 times. In June 1991, Stephen Findlay was found guilty of manslaughter by reason of diminished responsibility and was made the subject of a Hospital Order with restrictions on discharge (ss.37/41, Mental Health Act 1983).

The terms of reference of the Inquiry, set up in June 1991, were to:

- review the circumstances relating to the admission into Garlands Hospital and subsequent care, detention and discharge of Stephen Findley, and the procedures that were involved;
- review the investigations by the Unit General Manager and the Director of Public Health;
- consider the need for further investigations and, where appropriate, instigate action;
- inquire into the managerial action after the event;
- make recommendations to the Health Authority.

The report was published in October 1991 by the East Cumbria Health Authority and is available from the North Cumbria Health Authority, Wavell Drive, Rosehill, Carlisle CA1 2ST.

1990

REPORT OF THE INQUIRY INTO THE CIRCUMSTANCES LEADING TO THE DEATH IN BROADMOOR HOSPITAL OF JOSEPH WATTS

D Atha, Dr Christopher Hunter, K Newton, T Williams and David Downham CBE

Joseph Watts was born in Jamaica in 1958 and came to England when he was 2 years old. He was convicted of indecent assault in 1984 and admitted under ss.37/41, Mental Health Act 1983 to Broadmoor Hospital. He was placed in a seclusion room on 23rd August 1988 and subsequently injected with 200mg of Chlorpromazine. Within 2 minutes of the room being vacated, he was seen to be motionless. Staff re-entered the room and attempts at resuscitation were unsuccessful.

The terms of reference of the Inquiry were to:

- enquire into the circumstances leading to the death of Joseph Watts on 23rd August 1988, having regard to treatment plans since his admission to Broadmoor Hospital in 1984, dealing with his physical and mental health;
- consider the adequacy of the procedures for handling patients in a disturbed state;
- recommend any action that should be taken in patient care.

The report was completed in July 1989 and made public by the Special Hospitals Service Authority in June 1990.

REPORT OF THE PANEL OF INQUIRY APPOINTED BY THE NORTH STAFFORDSHIRE HEALTH AUTHORITY TO INVESTIGATE THE CIRCUMSTANCES OF THE DEATH OF ALMA SIMPSON

Jeffrey Burke QC, Eric Crossfield, Dr Edward Gordon, Dr James Higgins and Alexander Taylor

Alma Simpson was born in 1932. She was an in-patient at St. Edward's Hospital in 1951 and again in 1955 suffering from a psychiatric illness diagnosed originally as primary dementia and later as schizophrenia. She was admitted, usually informally, on twelve occasions between 1982 and her final admission on 28th May 1988.

She suffered a number of assaults from other patients and was also the perpetrator of a number of assaults. As a result of the assaults on her, her husband, complained to the hospital staff and management of his fears for his wife's safety on Ward 2. He made similar complaints to the local M.P. These fears turned out to be well-founded. During the evening of 31st May 1988, Alma Simpson, was found unconscious in a corridor on that ward. She had been brutally assaulted by another patient. She sustained injuries so serious that, despite surgery and intensive medical care, she died, aged 53, at the North Staffordshire Royal Infirmary on 6th June 1988.

The terms of reference of the Inquiry were originally as follows -

"The North Staffordshire Health Authority have received a complaint from Frederick Simpson arising out of an assault on his wife on 31st May 1988 while a patient on Ward 2, St. Edward's Hospital, Leek, Staffordshire, which assault occasioned her death. For the purpose of investigating this complaint within the procedure provided for in Circular HM(66)15 the Committee is requested to conduct a full investigation and, after investigating, to report to the North Staffordshire Health Authority, into the following matters insofar as they relate to the death of Alma Simpson:

- Any policy and/or general practice as to admissions of patients to St. Edward's Hospital and in particular Ward 2 at that Hospital;
- Any policy and/or general practice as to transfer of patients from Ward 2 to other wards at St. Edward's Hospital or to other hospitals;
- The staffing of Ward 2 between 1st March 1987 and 31st May 1988;
- The levels of violence exhibited by patients on Ward 2 between 1st March 1987 and 31st May 1988.
- The policy and arrangements relating to the care of violent patients on Ward 2 and in St. Edward's Hospital and other hospitals, if any, to which Alma Simpson might have been transferred;
- The circumstances surrounding the admission of Alma Simpson to Ward 2 on 28th May 1988;
- The circumstances surrounding the incident involving Alma Simpson on 31st May 1988 which led to her death."

In the course of the hearings it became clear that they could not fairly investigate the circumstances surrounding Alma Simpson's death without adding to the terms of reference; it was agreed by all parties that they had power to make such additions; on 4th October 1989 (Day 18), after hearing arguments from the parties, they exercised that power by adding the following to the terms of reference:-

- The treatment given to Alma Simpson at St. Edward's Hospital between 25th February 1987 and 31st May 1988;
- What diagnosis was made of her condition while she was on Menzies Ward between 25th February 1987 and 13th November 1987;
- What programme of treatment was devised while she was on Menzies Ward between 25th February 1987 and 13th November 1987;
- Whether, had a suitable programme of treatment been devised for and given during her admission to Menzies House after 25th February 1987 her behaviour would have been such that she would not have been transferred to Ward 2 on 13th November 1987 or admitted to Ward 2 during 1988;

- What diagnosis was made of her condition while she was on Ward 2 between 24th November 1987 and 31st May 1988;
- What programme of treatment was devised while she was on Ward 2 between 24th November 1987 and 31st May 1988;
- Whether she had a suitable programme of treatment been devised for and given during her admissions to Ward 2 after 24th November 1987 her behaviour would have been such that she would not have been on Ward 2 on 31st May 1988."

The report was published by the West Midlands Regional Health Authority in July 1990.

1988

REGIONAL FACT FINDING COMMITTEE OF INQUIRY: CARE AND TREATMENT OF PSYCHIATRIC PATIENTS IN NORTH LINCOLNSHIRE

Cyril Unwin MBE, P Hughes OBE, A Monahan, Dr D Morgan, Dr A Pattie

During the period 1st January 1985 to 17th July 1986, a number of deaths (13 by suicide, 2 accidental, 1 case of misadventure and 2 open verdicts) occurred among patients of St John's Hospital, Lincoln. They were aged between 25 and 79 and were mainly in-patients with the others attending as out-patients or day patients.

The terms of reference of the Inquiry, set up in August 1986, were to:

- enquire into the care and treatment of psychiatric patients in North Lincolnshire in the light of the recent deaths by suicide and accident of patients under the care of St John's Hospital, Lincoln, and to make recommendations.

A shortened version of the Committee of Inquiry's report was published by Trent Regional Health Authority in October 1988.

REPORT OF THE COMMITTEE OF INQUIRY INTO THE CARE AND AFTER-CARE OF SHARON CAMPBELL

John Spokes QC, Dr Michael Pare and George Royle

Isabel Schwarz, a social worker employed by Bexley SSD was killed at her office in Bexley Hospital on 6th July 1984. This followed telephone threat(s) in March 1984 by Sharon Campbell (then aged 22), a client of hers from September 1982 until October 1983. Sharon Campbell appeared in Court a year later and her plea of guilty to manslaughter on the ground of diminished responsibility was accepted at the Old Bailey and she was sent to Broadmoor Hospital under ss.37/41, Mental Health Act 1983. Pressure from Dr Victor Schwarz finally led to an Inquiry into the death of his daughter being established.

The terms of reference of the Inquiry, set up in March 1987, were to:

- inquire into the management of arrangements for the care and after-care of Sharon Campbell;
- consider the adequacy of these arrangements;
- report to the Secretary of State and to make recommendations, on the basis of their findings, on any measure or practices which might provide improvements in identifying the needs of mentally disordered people and in the quality of care for those living in the community and the support for staff working with them.

The report was published in July 1988 by HMSO - price £8.30.

1985

REPORT TO THE SECRETARY OF STATE FOR SOCIAL SERVICES CONCERNING THE DEATH OF MICHAEL MARTIN AT BROADMOOR HOSPITAL

Shirley Ritchie QC, Dr J Higgins, and C McLoughlin

Michael Martin was born in 1961. He first came to the attention of the psychiatric services in 1976. In June 1978 he was detained in Bexley Hospital under s.26, Mental Health Act 1959 and in November 1979 transferred to Broadmoor Hospital. He was placed in a seclusion room on 6th July 1984 and given an injection of 500mg of Sodium Amytal and 200mg of Sparine. Michael Martin was found dead in the seclusion room less than 2 hours later.

The terms of reference of the Inquiry were to:

- inquire into the circumstances surrounding the incident on 6th July 1984 involving Michael Martin, a patient at Broadmoor Hospital, following which he was found dead;
- consider the care and treatment accorded to Michael Martin before and during his seclusion on 6th July;
- report conclusions relating to this matter;
- and in the light of those conclusions recommend any action that should be taken in relation to patient care.

The report was published by the DHSS in 1985.

Sandhill Park Hospital Inquiry (1981)

This followed the resignation of a Sister, who was subsequently struck off the Register by the General Nursing Council, at this hospital for those with a learning disability in Somerset. The inquiry found 'no clear evidence that any overt cruelty was involved nor any indication that physical harm befell any patient'.

Newchurch Hospital Inquiry (1980)

This inquiry in Cheshire followed events in late 1978 which resulted in the conviction and imprisonment of a member of staff for the 'ill-treatment of patients'.

Cotshill Hospital Inquiry (1980)

This followed the conviction of a nursing assistant for assaulting patients with a mop. She was sentenced to imprisonment and two other staff faced disciplinary proceedings. Oxford Area Health Authority initiated a review of its services for those with a learning disability.

Brookwood Hospital Inquiry (1980)

An inquiry into Industrial Relations reported in 1979. This inquiry, set up by West Surrey/North East Hampshire Health District, into patient care considered allegations of violence, the lax over-administration of drugs and ill-treatment of patients.

Rampton Hospital Review (1980)

In May 1979, Yorkshire Television screened a programme, *The Secret Hospital*, where it alleged large-scale brutality involving a total of 801 cases. Well over 100 nurses were said to have been named by ex-patients as having been responsible.

St Mary's Hospital, Stannington, Inquiry (1979)

This inquiry by Gateshead Area Health Authority was into mainly administrative difficulties.

Winterton Hospital Inquiry (1979)

This followed a leaving presentation/party for a Sister at this large mental illness hospital in County Durham which led to an elderly lady being secluded all night "contrary to agreed nursing practice and the hospital policy on seclusion".

Church Hill House Hospital Inquiry (1979)

This inquiry at a Berkshire Hospital for those with a learning disability was mainly concerned with allegations of victimisation of members of one trade union by members of another but staff made various allegations of mistreatment of patients, lack of control of drugs and misuse of patients' funds. The police investigated these complaints but no charges were preferred. In July 1982 4 members of staff were given prison sentences for 'sadistic acts of violence' committed during the period December 1980 and June 1981 (i.e. starting not much more than a year after the publication of the inquiry report).

Rainhill Hospital Inquiry (1979)

This was set up by Liverpool Area Health Authority to "review industrial relations and allegations of irregularities and malpractice's."

Normansfield Hospital Inquiry (1978)

This inquiry followed a strike by nurses for nearly nine hours. It heard evidence on 124 days and the transcript ran to 15,000 pages and examined events of the preceding five and a half years and centred upon the behaviour of the Consultant Psychiatrist in Subnormality whose contract the inquiry recommended should be immediately terminated and he should not be "re-engaged in any capacity in the National Health Service".

Mary Dendy Hospital Inquiry (1977)

This inquiry was into the management of this hospital in Cheshire for people with a learning disability where there were instances of bad nursing practice.

Warlingham Park Hospital Inquiry (1976)

This inquiry into a mental illness hospital was set up by Croydon Area Health Authority following concern aroused by the apparently high number of suicides by in-patients and out-patients in a 17 month period during 1974 and 1975.

Darlington Memorial Hospital Inquiry (1976)

This inquiry was set up by the Northern Regional Health Authority in 1975 to investigate the deaths of 4 patients in the psychiatric unit at the hospital in Newcastle who had died within a period of 5 weeks in the summer of 1975. There was no ill-treatment but there were suggestions of inadequate staffing, poor nursing management, administrative complacency about fire precautions, and generally unsatisfactory management at unit level.

St Augustine's Hospital Inquiry (1976)

This report was published by the South East Thames Regional Health Authority into conditions on the long-stay wards at St Augustine's Hospital, near Canterbury between 1972 and 1975.

Psychiatric Department, Bolton General Hospital (1976)

This followed a complaint of unlawful detention and also examined "the behaviour of hospital staff towards patients".

St Ebba's Hospital Inquiry (1975)

This report by Merton, Sutton and Wandsworth Area Health Authority followed a scalding accident.

South Ockendon Hospital Inquiry (1974)

This followed the death of an 18 year old male patient in 1969 at this hospital for patients with a learning disability on the eastern outskirts of London and the resignation of a State Enrolled Nurse in 1972 who made "serious allegations of unprofessional conduct and low nursing standards against one of the charge nurses". The committee started work in May 1972 and submitted its report the following March but it was not published until May 1974.

Inquiry into the death of Daniel Carey at Tooting Bec Hospital (1974)

Daniel Carey, aged 52, was a State Enrolled Nurse who had worked at Tooting Bec Hospital for 20 years. He was stabbed to death at the hospital on 2nd August 1974 by Samuel Hall, an informal patient. Samuel Hall had a diagnosis of schizophrenia and, since 1963, had been admitted on several occasions to hospital, including periods whilst detained under the Mental Health Act 1959. He had been a patient at Tooting Bec Hospital since March 1967. In April 1974, a sheath knife and 4 pen knives had been found under his bed by a nurse and removed. The report was published by South West Thames RHA.

Napsbury Hospital Report (1973)

The Secretary of State for Social Services set up this "professional investigation" following an unusual number of complaints concerning patient care at this North London Hospital. This included the death of a patient who at a post-mortem examination was found to have suffered severe and extensive injuries which may have been caused by a road accident some days before her death and which had not been noticed whilst a patient on the ward. The inquiry also commented on the crisis intervention service and the unorthodox methods of one Consultant Psychiatrist who had managed to achieve "good results in a notoriously difficult group of patients".

Whittingham Hospital Inquiry (1972)

Two senior members of staff at this long stay hospital in Lancashire complained directly to the Secretary of State for Social Services alleging "ill-treatment of patients, fraud and maladministration, including suppression of complaints from student nurses". The focus was on 4 wards with one ward, under the supervision of a Sister who had worked in it continuously for 47 years, being particularly bad.

Farleigh Hospital Inquiry (1971)

This followed a police investigation which led to 9 nurses at this hospital in Bristol for men with a learning disability being charged with offences relating to cruelty. 6 were acquitted but 3 were found guilty and received sentences of several years' imprisonment. The inquiry did not investigate the ill-treatment of patients any further but concentrated on the 'administration of and conditions at the hospital ... particularly as they were during the period July 1967 to December 1968 when the offences were committed'.

Ely Hospital Inquiry (1969)

This followed a Nursing Assistant at Ely Hospital, Cardiff making a series of specific allegations in 1967 to the *News of the World* about the treatment of patients and the pilfering of property by staff members. The hospital cared for approximately 600 patients, of whom the majority were considered to have a learning disability. An inquiry was set up under Sir Geoffrey Howe QC to examine allegations of cruel ill-treatment of 4 particular patients by 6 named members of staff, generally inhumane and threatening behaviour towards patients by one staff member, pilfering of food, clothing and other items belonging to the hospital or the patients, indifference on the part of the Chief Male Nurse to complaints that were made to him and lack of care by the Physician Superintendent and one other member of the medical staff.

The report criticised individual nurses of 'old-fashioned and unsophisticated techniques' of control but found that in most instances the ill-treatment was not due to 'wilful or malicious misconduct'.

SELECTED CONCERNS AND RECOMMENDATIONS FROM INQUIRIES PUBLISHED BETWEEN 1985 - 1996

PSYCHIATRIC SERVICES - General

- Key workers under the Care Programme Approach should only be eligible for appointment when they are competent to:
  - **i)** identify and record symptoms which may represent significant risk;
  - **ii)** discuss these immediately with their supervisors or an experienced worker;
  - **iii)** convey their concerns to a consultant psychiatrist or other doctor approved under s.12, Mental Health Act 1983 *(Sinclair p.77)*.

- Mental Health Care must be given a higher priority within the Trust and the Health Authority *(Hampshire p.70)*.

- The Chair of the Trust and the Chair of the Health Authority must make a joint visit to Gregory Ward to see for themselves the unacceptable conditions to which patients are being admitted *(Hampshire p.70)*.

- The Health Authority, in conjunction with other local agencies, must take steps to secure radical improvements to Mental Health services. The following should be taken into account:
  - **(a)** the implications of the new Mental Health (Patients in the Community) Act 1995;
  - **(b)** the NHS Executive Guidance on the Care Programme Approach and the development of a spectrum of mental health services;
  - **(c)** the adverse observations about mental health services within the area made over several years by the Mental Health Act Commission and the local Community Health Council;
  - **(d)** the lack of community facilities and alternatives to in-patient care;
  - **(e)** the deplorable state of Gregory Ward *(Hampshire p.70)*.

- The Trust should ensure that all members of the clinical psychiatric team (at all levels) have access to proper clinical supervision, preferably entirely independent of their own workload. We do not consider the present arrangements (monthly formal meetings between the consultant psychiatrist and the Community Psychiatric Nurse team manager and informal discussions between the treating doctors and the Community Psychiatric Nurses at weekly ward rounds) to be adequate *(Hampshire p.71)*.

- Anger management therapy should only be undertaken by or under the close supervision of experienced qualified staff. Failure of this form of treatment should lead to a consideration of alternative treatments including referral to a specialist centre *(Gadher p.29)*.

- Consideration should be given to the development of a discrete personal care service *(Viner p.42)*.

- If closure of a case occurs, this must be handled with sensitivity and with due regard by the agency responsible to the possible outcome of such an action on the person *(Southampton p.10)*.

- Keyworkers are responsible for ensuring that proposed interventions, eg outpatient appointments, are organised and for monitoring them *(Southampton p.10)*.

- Consideration should be given to adequate staff protection and support when dealing with certain clients. The particular history of the client and experience/characteristics of professional personnel should always be taken into account *(Southampton p.10).*

- Keyworkers must personally undertake an assessment and maintain appropriate direct contact with allocated clients *(Southampton p.10).*

- Personality disorder in its own right should not be used as a criterion for acceptance or rejection from the team's services, but other indicators of severity and disability associated with mental health problems should be applied, including psychiatric history *(Southampton p.10).*

- In allocating cases the team manager must have regard both to the complexity of the case and to the experience and skills of the worker *(Southampton p.10).*

- Services need to recognise that patients may find multiple points of access confusing *(Southampton p.10).*

- Engagement with services needs to be tailored to the individual client. Thus for clients who are reluctant to leave home, out-patients' appointments may be ineffectual *(Southampton p.10).*

- There should be a continuing education and training programme set up to inform medical, nursing, management and social services staff about the Mental Health Act 1983, in particular the legal status and rights of patients admitted and detained under one of its sections. Given the frequency of transfers to Hackney Hospital from prison, special emphasis should be placed on the ramifications of those sections which deal with the transfer to hospital from court or prison *(Grey p.49).*

- A firm commitment should be given to the joint commissioning of services for people with severe mental health needs, in the first instance for younger adults (16 to 64 years of age), and agree upon a joint strategy for future provision where the primary emphasis is on prevention, care and aftercare in the community *(Woodley p.162).*

- In the process of collaboration with joint commissioning, statutory authority purchasers take a needs-led, rather than service-led approach *(Woodley p.162).*

- Aggregate budgets for older people, younger adults and children should be taken into account when determining financial allocation on the basis of priority need, and in so doing, determine whether virement is appropriate and possible in order to meet shortfalls for people who have serious mental health needs *(Woodley p.162).*

- Local social services authorities and district health authorities should, when publishing Community Care Plans on services for people with mental health needs, identify the number, sex, age and ethnicity, together with need profiles of inpatients in specialist psychiatric services as well as people living in the community, so that the totality of services, location and future needs of all service users are included *(Woodley p.163).*

- The North West London Mental Health NHS Trust should ensure that all new patients referred to the Outpatients Clinic are seen by or discussed with the Consultant or Senior Registrar and that the resulting formulation is clearly recorded in the case notes and communicated to the GP *(Boland p.29).*

- The Trust should ensure that it becomes standard procedure for outpatients carried by a junior doctor to be discussed with the Consultant when the junior doctor comes to the end of his or her placement with the team. A review and possible reformulation of the patient's problems should be recorded in the case notes. At the least, a handover note should be made in the case notes describing the salient problems for the junior doctor who next takes over the case *(Boland p.29)*.

- The Trust should ensure that, if patients are kept on in the Outpatients Clinic primarily for the purpose of being recruited into a drug trial, the proposition should be discussed and agreed with the patient, the patient's GP and the local ethical committee *(Boland p.30)*.

- The Trust should ensure that a review takes place to establish a standard procedure for recording important messages received e.g. by daily log *(Boland p.30)*.

- Even the most skilled and experienced amongst us can benefit from reflecting on our practice under the guidance of a skilled practitioner whom we trust. Within social work and psychotherapy, this is a well established practice. For nursing, it has long been a feature of community work. It is rapidly gaining ground in other settings. Working in Partnership recommends 'that new training initiatives aimed at developing clinical supervision skills in senior clinical nurses are devised. We also recommend that newly qualified nurses and nursing students receive preparation in what to expect from clinical supervision'. We would fully support that recommendation, and would further support the extension of the principle to all mental health professionals of all grades *(The Falling Shadow p.140)*.

- We strongly endorse the importance of a personal visit from a member of staff (to the victim of a delusional obsession), to assess the truth of the allegations and to hear at first hand the facts of the problem. The key worker, the responsible Community Psychiatric Nurse or team social worker, would be ideally placed to make such a visit ... No breach of confidentiality will normally be involved in receiving and assessing information, but, if there is a clear risk to a member of the public, then there is an over-riding duty to breach confidence and to provide information in so far as it is necessary in the interests of the potential victim *(The Falling Shadow p.149)*.

- The British Medical Association recommends that consultant job plans should at most contain five fixed sessions so that the remaining sessions may be used in a more flexible fashion. We would particularly recommend the freeing up of more time for liaison, community visits and communication with professionals who are unable to attend Ward Rounds *(Dalson p.15)*.

- There should be multi-agency discussions between Health, Social Services, Police Service, representatives of ethnic minorities and all other parties with an interest in looking at issues around the use of cannabis and how those vulnerable to its effects may be protected *(Dalson p.15)*.

- Policies and procedures need to offer a reliable and usable framework of guidance for staff to draw upon in their daily work *(Thameside p.26)*.

- Contacts with the media need to be cultivated *(S.Devon p.87)*.

- Each psychiatric service should actively recruit medical practitioners to make certain that there are sufficient doctors in their area who are approved under s.12, Mental Health Act 1983 to ensure prompt response to requests for assessment under the Act *(Clunis p.129)*.

- We suggest that urgent requests should be met within 3 hours and non-urgent requests within 3 working days. The performance of these targets must be properly monitored *(Clunis p.129)*.

- Setting up a rota of s.12 approved doctors available at all times to visit patients in the catchment area with ASW's to assess whether compulsory admission is necessary *(NW London p.41)*.

- Agreement with accident and emergency departments policies for assessment and admission of patients to psychiatric wards. The policies should include specifications for: nursing supervision of patients while in the accident and emergency department, (including the interval between psychiatric assessment and admission), more effective supervision of junior medical staff, and prompt attendance of a senior doctor approved under s.12, Mental Health Act 1983, when compulsory admission is contemplated *(NW London p.41)*.

- Management should ensure adequate opportunities for on-going development of the professional skills of all members of care teams *(Oxfordshire p.7)*.

- The head of mental health nursing should:
  - ▲ set a programme with targets and deadlines for the further on-going development and enhancement of nursing care plans;
  - ▲ establish a training programme to clarify and re-define the criteria and threshold for nurse calls for medical assistance in the unit. Multi-professional commitment to this programme will be required;
  - ▲ provide guidelines about nursing handover arrangements at weekends and for inter-ward transfer;
  - ▲ review the present systems available for the supervision and training of nursing staff *(Shrodells p.8)*.

- The layout, design and use of the unit and the levels of medical and nurse staffing should be examined to ensure safe standards of care *(Shrodells p.8)*.

- The Mental Health Act Code of Practice should be adopted as the framework to set safe standards for the mental health service. Explicit requirements will include a review of facilities to receive patients detained under s.136, Mental Health Act 1983 and a review of the present policies for the admission of patients to the unit. To ensure that these are effective, a review of the present arrangements for the on-going training and counselling of staff will be required *(Shrodells p.8)*.

- Where appropriate external expert assistance is provided for training and counselling of all staff *(Shrodells p.10)*.

  a) There should be a comprehensive survey of needs and services within the community and the determination of an up-to-date strategy and structure to meet those needs.
  b) The role of the team and its individual members should be carefully and clearly defined.
  c) There should be clear procedures for the effective liaison and communication between the different disciplines within each team and with hospital based services.
  d) An adequate system for monitoring and evaluating the delivery of services will be required.
  e) Perhaps every patient, and certainly every patient who is or has recently been seriously disturbed, should not leave the hospital either on discharge or on extended leave until there has, within the last month or other suitable period, been a case conference involving all the disciplines appropriate to the patient's case, including the appropriate community team; the purpose of such a conference should be to facilitate informed discussion and decision on whether the patient should be in the community or should remain in hospital, on the assessment of and a treatment plan for the patient's future needs in the community, medical and social, and on the provision to be made to meet those needs. This system may not always

be possible in the case of informal patients who choose to discharge themselves before such a case conference has been convened; short of regular case conferences for all cases, it is difficult to know how to meet such cases; consideration should be given to developing a system which will meet them.
f) Consideration should be given to establishing the principle of a case manager from within the appropriate team for each case involving a patient who is or has recently been seriously mentally ill, analogously with the key worker principle operating within the hospital wards *(Simpson p 108)*.

- Steps should be taken to re-align sectors in the Mental Health Unit to correspond with Local Authority Social Services boundaries *(N.Lincolnshire p.iii)*.

- Appropriate education and training should be provided for all staff involved with new psychodynamic approaches *(N.Lincolnshire p.iv)*.

- Continuing education and training regarding the provisions of the Mental Health Act 1983 (and related procedures) should be provided for all staff concerned *(N.Lincolnshire p.vi)*.

- More informal links should be developed and maintained with the local media. Appropriate steps should be taken to ensure that confidential information concerning patients is safeguarded *(N.Lincolnshire p.ix)*.

- A formal policy concerning links with the media (including clarification of which officers are designated as spokespersons) should be issued *(N.Lincolnshire p.ix)*.

- Appropriate use of professional public relations expertise should be made *(N.Lincolnshire p.ix)*.

- The use of negative or "no comment" statements when responding to questions from the media should be avoided *(N.Lincolnshire p.ix)*.

- Greater support should be given to junior medical staff in their clinical work *(N.Lincolnshire p.xi)*.

- All entries in medical and nursing records should be written legibly *(N.Lincolnshire p.xii)*.

PSYCHIATRIC SERVICES - Multi-disciplinary working

- Communications within a multi-disciplinary team are fostered when there is a constant membership. The social work membership of the Hartlepool Team is not currently constituted like that and we recommend that their functioning is continually audited and altered in line with other Cleveland Community Mental Health Teams if considered necessary *(Armstrong p.98)*.

- More direct action should be taken to ensure that referrals to Drug and Alcohol Agencies are made and that the initiative is not left to the patient alone. It is however, accepted that individual patient commitment and responsibility is equally important *(Armstrong p.99)*.

- If a patient has missed more than 2 outpatient appointments, the clinical team must follow up to establish the reason for such non-attendance *(Hampshire p.71)*.

- Any proper care plan must contain a contingency plan to be put into effect in the event of the failure of the primary plan. A multi-agency case conference should be held if the situation is complex enough to warrant it *(Hampshire p.72)*.

- All relevant clinical information about the patient should be passed between the treating psychiatrists, the GP, the Community Psychiatric Nurse and Social Services, where involved *(Hampshire p.72)*.

- All persons known to suffer from severe mental disorder should continue to receive appropriate support from a multidisciplinary Mental Health Team and should not be expected to rely on the duty social worker for assistance *(Gadher p.26)*.

- All statutory, voluntary and independent agencies (particularly including GP's) likely to be involved in the care of patients subject to the Care Programme Approach procedure should be invited to attend Care Programme Approach meetings and should receive copies of the record of the meeting whether they attend or not *(Gadher p.31)*.

- As well as the user, all likely carers of patients subject to the Care Programme Approach procedure should be invited to attend Care Programme Approach meetings and should receive copies of the record of the meeting whether they attend or not *(Gadher p.31)*.

- The Care Programme Approach documentation should include information as to the nature of the patient's medication (at least indicating whether it is taken orally or by depot injection). In line with the recommendations made in other Inquiry Reports, we recommend that all members of the team should be alerted to the signs and symptoms in the patient which may indicate that the patient is likely to relapse. These indications may be identified by the doctors, the patient or carers. Non compliance with medication should be recognised as a significant pointer to a relapse *(Gadher p.33)*.

- A deputy for the key worker should be identified and the identity recorded at the Care Programme Approach meeting and the key worker and deputy should not be on holiday together without making specific arrangements for cover. These should include arrangements for handover and for notification to all concerned *(Gadher p.33)*.

- Out-patient reviews of patients subject to the Care Programme Approach procedure should be under the close supervision of the responsible consultant and doctors without the qualification MRCPsych should not assess patients except under supervision *(Gadher p.34)*.

- The Trust and SSD develop a costed and timescaled strategic plan for the development and implementation of integrated multidisciplinary Community and Mental Health Teams as soon as is practicable *(Gadher p.36)*.

- Professional supervision and managerial support should be readily available to Community Mental Health Centre and Team Managers. Community Psychiatric Nurse caseloads should be kept under review and Community Psychiatric Nurse record keeping should be subjected to an internal audit process *(Gadher p.36)*.

- All personnel having to do with the operation of the Mental Health Act should be reminded at the earliest possible opportunity that the words used in ss.2 and 3 of the Act are "health *or* safety" and not "health *and* safety" *(Gadher p.38)*.

- The Medical Director of the Trust in consultation with the medical staff and with their agreement should implement a policy whereby consultants and junior doctors should so arrange their leave that no more than one medical member of a team is away at any one time. A consultant who is going on leave should ensure that the key worker for all patients subject to the Care Programme Approach procedure is aware of the arrangements made for cover *(Gadher p.38).*

- The Medical Director of the Trust should formulate and circulate a clear policy statement indicating the circumstances in which it would be appropriate for professional staff to notify the Driver and Vehicle Licensing Agency of the illness of a patient *(Gadher p.40).*

- Consideration should be given to the desirability of including in the Care Programme Approach documentation a note of the advice given to the patient about driving *(Gadher p.41).*

- Acute Occupational Therapy staff are now integrated into the Community Mental Health Team's. However the rehabilitation Occupational Therapy service remains separate both from the acute Occupational Therapy service and from the Community Mental Health Teams. All agencies need to have a clear understanding of the role of the rehabilitation Occupational Therapy service and bringing the services professionally closer would promote a more efficient service *(Viner p.23).*

- Any referral by a Care Programme Approach keyworker for a specific service from another agency should be confirmed in writing and a copy of any care plan should be made available *(Viner p.40).*

- The social services department should examine the linkages within the service, in particular those between the rehabilitation and mental health teams, and provide guidance to staff on the need to take into account the potential for onward referral between the teams *(Viner p.41).*

- All health professionals, who are going to have to undertake a key worker role under the Care Programme Approach, should be involved in joint multi-agency training with housing and social services staff. The purpose of the training would be to broaden the understanding of the function and role of these two agencies in the accommodation field and to further their understanding of the resources available *(Viner p.41).*

- An inter-agency confidentiality policy should be developed which must include reference to the carer's circumstances *(Viner p.52).*

- Greater consideration of the use of guardianship under the Mental Health Act 1983 should be given to cases where individuals with long term mental health problems are being supported in the community but are opposed to moving to alternative accommodation. This will require comprehensive multi-agency training *(Viner p.59).*

- Consideration should be given to establishing protocols and procedures for screening all Care Programme Approach cases. This is to ensure that the lead agency/authority in a Care Programme Approach case can evaluate whether the statutory or other duties and obligations imposed on other agencies/authorities are being fulfilled. Similarly, if another agency/authority is asked to assist then that organisation can assess if the request is compatible with their own statutory or other duties *(Viner p.59).*

- Multi-agency training should be arranged to allow health professionals, who are likely to be keyworkers under the Care Programme Approach, to understand the resources and legal obligations of social services departments and housing agencies. The legal obligations that are imposed on local authorities in relation to provision for carers should be a matter for particular attention *(Viner p.60).*

- Care plans must be made available to agencies and workers to whom a referral has been made for involvement in mental health care *(Viner p.65).*

- Consideration needs to be given to the agencies establishing a process for resolving any disagreement that may arise over the implementation of a care plan *(Viner p.65).*

- In line with national guidance which requires that the Care Programme Approach is applied to all mentally ill patients who are accepted by the specialist mental health services, existing local joint policy/procedural guidelines on the Care Programme Approach should be reviewed, to identify the Care Programme Approach tiers that will be operated locally and to define entry requirements to those tiers with as much precision as possible *(Viner p.65).*

- Consideration should be given to the promotion of inter-agency and inter-disciplinary relationships within the Community Mental Health Teams. Particular attention should be paid to the management of Community Mental Health Team's in order to assist the teams to function effectively as integrated units *(Viner p.75).*

- Attention should be given to the development and implementation of a supervision policy for all mental health professionals, including doctors, of all grades. Also any policy must make explicit the mechanisms that will ensure that every current case managed by a professional is automatically reviewed within a specified period *(Viner p.79).*

- Significant contributions to clinical assessments by professional staff in disciplines other than psychiatry and nursing should be captured systematically, e.g. in the compilation of reports for case conferences, other reviews and hospital transfers *(Mitchell p.42).*

- Where there are a number of services or agencies involved in the care and treatment of an individual, consideration needs to be given as to which has the lead role in what circumstances *(Southampton p.10).*

- Where there are specialist social workers in the Community Mental Health Team, all social services interventions for potential Community Mental Health Team clients should be via that team rather than via the Social Services Area Centre *(Southampton p.11).*

- Where non-specialist (ie. non mental health) agencies are the only link with a client, they should have agreed criteria with specialist agencies for referral and re-referral *(Southampton p.11).*

- Non mental health agencies should never be left without some degree of specialist backup, co-ordinated by a joint working plan, unless it is agreed as unnecessary *(Southampton p.11).*

- All information essential to effective care planning should be exchanged between the in-patient and community services in a timely fashion. This should be the subject of rigorous joint monitoring and audit by health and social services *(Southampton p.11).*

- Where parallel processes occur (e.g. hospital and Community Mental Health Team reviews) agencies need to inform each other prior to reviews taking place *(Southampton p.11).*

- The Community Mental Health Team must be involved in, and agree to, the discharge planning *(Southampton p.11)*.

- The clarification of responsibilities in regard to inter-agency communication should be seen as a priority by all relevant agencies *(Southampton p.11)*.

- Local managers must review mechanisms for resolving inter-agency policy disputes *(Southampton p.11)*.

- Information systems need to be established to allow the discovery of existing and recent service links of people with mental health problems living in the community, while not ignoring confidentiality issues *(Southampton p.11)*.

- While health and social services have to play their part as the joint agencies responsible for care in the community, they can only operate in partnership with other agencies and those living in the community *(Southampton p.11)*.

- A link should be established between the patient and a member of the Mental Health Locality Team from the time of admission until the time a Key Worker is allocated if a Key worker is considered necessary *(Grey p.51)*.

- Any involvement of any member of the Mental Health Locality Team should be construed as a referral to the team as a whole and should be logged immediately *(Grey p.51)*.

- The Mental Health Locality Team (and the Probation Service where already involved) should be informed immediately on the patient's admission to hospital under section *(Grey p.49)*.

- The importance of team working between hospital, community and primary care needs emphasis and constant review *(Doherty - N.Ireland p.79)*.

- A compatible information system between mental health and social services should be established to facilitate greater continuity of care *(Doherty - N.Ireland p.82)*.

- All staff likely to use powers under the Mental Health (NI) Order 1986 should have received induction training in its use. Training should include full knowledge of the additional guidance contained in the Guide to the Order and the Code of Practice. In addition there should be regular refresher training *(Doherty - N.Ireland p.83)*.

- All staff likely to use powers under the Mental Health (NI) Order 1986 should have ready access to legal advice concerning any aspects where they are unsure of the interpretation *(Doherty - N.Ireland p.83)*.

- Social services and district health authorities should jointly assess their training needs and develop joint training strategies to promote multidisciplinary working arrangements for Care in the Community, in conjunction with service users and housing and voluntary organisations *(Woodley p.109)*.

- Local social services authorities and district health authorities should pool their mental health training resources in order to promote and target multi-disciplinary training *(Woodley p.163)*.

- The NHS commissioning authority and Department of Social Services should make a joint plan which is then carried out to make provision for all severely mentally ill people living in their area. This should include provision for the homeless severely mentally ill for whom the high concentration of skills and professional training of the health provider Trust are particularly required. Access to services for the mentally ill, both within and outside normal working hours, both for routine and for emergency care, should be advertised to users, carers, other statutory bodies and voluntary agencies *(Newby p.151)*.

- The Health Authority and Social Services Authority should ensure that all such service providers are aware of the steps to be taken and the persons to contact in the event that an emergency assessment or admission to hospital appears necessary for a client. This information should be published and made widely available throughout the field of statutory and voluntary care, to carers themselves, to other agencies such as police and emergency services *(Newby p.153)*.

- The voluntary agencies, especially the Cyrenians, attempted to fill a gap in the provision of services - residential care for the homeless mentally ill. The Social Services Department of Oxfordshire County Council had not been involved either with the identifying of or providing for this deficiency in as much as the responsibility for finding accommodation for homeless mentally ill people had fallen on the Housing Department of the City of Oxford, a separate authority. Whereas the Health Authority would have provided comprehensive care for psychiatric in-patients, it would only give intermittent out-patient care via a consultant psychiatrist to a person whose key worker came from an independent voluntary organisation and whose accommodation was provided by another voluntary agency. There is clearly a need for much better organisation and integration for the care of individuals with severe mental illness. This might be achieved by clarifying the role and responsibilities of the Responsible Medical Officer in the community and ensuring that the resources including relevant trained personnel were available to do this *(Newby p.155)*.

- The Trust should ensure that, as part of the care plan, there are regular reviews of the progress of patients attending the Outpatients Clinic by senior doctors, if possible with other members of the multidisciplinary team, so that social and psychological dimensions can be identified and dealt with *(Boland p.29)*.

- The Trust should ensure that, where it is suspected that a social problem is significantly contributing to a patient's illness, the aetiology is pursued either by referral to social services or by establishing family work within the Outpatients Clinic. Thus, if a patient fails to respond to a particular line of care, other dimensions, including psycho-social dimensions, can be considered and explored by the multidisciplinary team *(Boland p.29)*.

- The Trust should undertake a project to consolidate and amalgamate the various sources of information, particularly separate sets of case notes, about patients attending different facilities *(Boland p.29)*.

- The Trust should urgently reappraise the roles of different staff members in relation to the discharge process. It may be appropriate for the key worker to co-ordinate and communicate the fact of discharge to the GP but this should be followed by a more detailed letter from the medical staff which should include a review of progress and the keyworker's impressions of the case *(Boland p.29)*.

- The Trust should ensure that the channels of communication between the medical teams and the Social Services Department are kept in good repair although there is no longer a social work attachment to medical teams. Whatever the details of delivery, they should be such that any client can be assessed by a social work care manager and appropriate arrangements made for them, post-assessment *(Boland p.30)*.

- As the patient progresses (and regresses) through the mental health system, there should go with him/her a full chronology *(The Falling Shadow p.38)*

- One step that could and should have been taken as a matter of urgency, was the abandonment of separate professional notes, and the development of multi-disciplinary records. At the same time as integrating professional notes into a single record, attention should be paid to integrating hospital and community records. The ideal to aim for is a single mental health record for each patient, irrespective of where they are treated, or by whom *(The Falling Shadow p.140)*.

- With current technology it would be straightforward in complex cases to have a thorough case summary which could be updated as new information became available. Such an extended summary could be passed on to future clinical teams *(The Falling Shadow p.180)*.

- The Trust should review the method of maintaining case notes on patients, with a view to holding multi-disciplinary records which are chronologically ordered to easily reflect the care afforded patients over time *(Buchanan p.23)*.

- Members of the multi-disciplinary team should be appropriately trained and experienced to deal with the client group involved *(Buchanan p.24)*.

- The multi-disciplinary working relationship between members of the team should be reviewed, particularly in respect to social work input *(Buchanan p.24)*.

- Brent Social Services Department should be asked to give careful consideration to the deployment, training and support of social workers and ensure that the most able and experienced staff are allocated to difficult and demanding patients *(Buchanan p.24)*.

- An agreed method of multidisciplinary assessment together with clear guidelines and standardised documentation should be introduced *(Usoro p.16)*.

- At the time of discharge from hospital or at change of residence, the community psychiatric service should notify the relevant GP as soon as s/he is known. This notification should include early contact with the GP by the community psychiatric service with regard to diagnosis, treatment programme, and the support to be provided by the community psychiatric service *(Usoro p.16)*.

- The work of Community Psychiatric Nurses should be more integrated within the day to day work of multidisciplinary community mental health team *(Inweh p.10)*.

- Changes in medication should be reported to Community Psychiatric Nurses and social workers covering a case *(Inweh p.11)*.

- A policy for reporting non-compliance with medication should be agreed between on the one hand, professional and voluntary staff working in the community, and, on the other, the prescribing doctors *(Inweh p.16)*.

- The management potential of senior doctors and nurses should be reviewed with the help of the Regional Director of Public Health and Regional Director of Nursing to ensure effective inter-disciplinary working and to maximise the management potential of these groups and others *(Shrodells p.7)*.

- Management of the Mental Health Unit should initiate a review into the effectiveness of communications between hospital staff, community psychiatric nurses, GP's and social workers. It is recognised that these relationships may improve as a result of the proposed sectorisation of mental health services *(Findlay p.18)*.

- There is a need to continue and enhance the progress which has been made towards the development of multi-disciplinary team working, particularly in a community context *(N.Lincolnshire p.v)*.

- Appropriate social work support should be provided for multi-disciplinary teams *(N.Lincolnshire p.v)*.

- Improvements in training and support for multi-disciplinary team working should be provided *(N.Lincolnshire p.v)*.

- The Unit Management Team should address the complex issues of accountability, responsibility etc. involved in multi-disciplinary work, thereby clarifying the framework for its operation in the Mental Health Unit *(N.Lincolnshire p.v)*.

- Decisions regarding support for patients (whether discharged from hospital or in the community) should be taken on a multi-disciplinary basis *(N.Lincolnshire p.xiii)*.

- Decisions regarding support for patients (whether discharged from hospital or in the community) should be taken on a multi-disciplinary basis *(N.Lincolnshire p.xiii)*.

PSYCHIATRIC SERVICES - Monitoring and inspection

- The recommended actions of the Trust's internal inquiry, i.e. that audit should occur and that reappointments should be within two months at the outside, ought to be implemented as soon as possible *(Armstrong p.99)*.

- The Health Authority and the Trust should continue to monitor the quality of the service and ensure that corrective action takes place *(Armstrong p.100)*.

- The joint commissioning agencies should review the current staff/population ratio of Community Mental Health Team staff *(Southampton p.10)*.

- The Care Programme Approach and supervision register arrangements in relation to the Community Mental Health Team must be reviewed *(Southampton p.11)*.

- Incident reporting needs to be systematised as part and parcel of professional practice. The system should be designed primarily for the direct benefit of management and staff, for the ultimate benefit of patient care. Only as a subsidiary purpose should it be designed to support a complaints system *(S.Devon p.85)*.

- Incidents should be kept under constant review by an Incident Review Committee established for the mental health service; and Mental Health Act Managers should be encouraged to review quarterly reports by the Committee to the Board of the Trust *(S.Devon p.85)*.

- A duty should be imposed on service providers in their contracts with commissioning authorities to satisfy an external inspecting or accrediting body that they have currently achieved published standards of service and facilities *(Clunis p.124)*.

- Need for the setting up of an annual audit of suicides *(NW London p.42)*.

- Mechanisms for the regular review of policies and procedures should be established and reports to be regularly provided to the District Health Authority *(Shrodells p.9)*.

- Routine monitoring should take place of rates of admission, readmission and of admissions under sections of the Mental Health Act 1983 *(N.Lincolnshire p.v)*.

- A review of communications, relationships and industrial relations should be undertaken in the Mental Health Unit *(N.Lincolnshire p.viii)*.

- Appropriate action should be taken to ensure that all Consultants comply with the requirements of the Mental Health Act *(N.Lincolnshire p.x)*.

PSYCHIATRIC SERVICES - Race and culture

- When allocating resources (finance, staffing, information, etc.) that proper account is taken of the different age structures within different ethnic groups in the district population, as well as socio-economic factors, and measures needed to be taken to eradicate institutional racism *(Woodley p.162)*.

- The statutory authorities serving Newham should actively promote the development of mental health service user forums throughout all services, together with an independent, ethnically sensitive advocacy service for people with severe mental health needs *(Woodley p.163)*.

- Broadmoor Hospitals' equal opportunities policy should deal with the problem of racism in the forensic psychiatric system as a whole and its effects within the hospital *(Blackwood p.78)*.

- Special Hospitals Service Authority, in conjunction with other relevant bodies, should give consideration to the commissioning of further research into the diagnosis of schizophrenia in Afro-Caribbean's *(Blackwood p.78)*.

- Special Hospitals Service Authority should monitor patterns of diagnosis among ethnic minority groups in the special hospital system *(Blackwood p.78)*.

- The monitoring of levels of medication should include an examination of how prescribing practices relate to the ethnic origins of patients *(Blackwood p.78)*.

- The Director of Personnel at Broadmoor Hospital should introduce stringent ethnic monitoring of the whole recruitment process *(Blackwood p.78)*.

- Special Hospitals Service Authority should consider revising its recruitment policy to ensure adequate opportunity for persons from the ethnic minority community to be appointed to senior management positions *(Blackwood p.79).*

- Special Hospitals Service Authority should consider the feasibility of establishing future high security facilities centred on a racially mixed, inner city area *(Blackwood p.79).*

- Occupational Therapy activities on the special care unit and elsewhere should address the clinical and personal needs of the individuals catered for, and in particular should be more culturally relevant *(Blackwood p.79).*

- The Director of Planning and Administration should ensure that a range of dietary choices are offered to patients, and should encourage diversity *(Blackwood p.79).*

- The location of community mental health centres should take account of the needs of ethnic communities *(Campbell p.77).*

- Training of health and social services staff should take account the importance of their being able to recognise and respond to the needs of people from differing cultural and ethnic backgrounds *(Campbell p.77).*

PSYCHIATRIC SERVICES - Gender

- In view of the level of disturbance of patients, the nature of their serious offences, and the vulnerability of women as a small minority group in a locked setting within the overall patient population, that a dedicated women-only ward be established within the new purpose built secure unit currently being commissioned to comply with the Department of Health's Patients' Charter *(Woodley p.51).*

- Health service providers should give serious consideration to the safety and needs of the small minority of women who are placed in secure health provision and to the need for choice of single sex wards in all psychiatric hospitals *(Woodley p.163).*

PSYCHIATRIC SERVICES - Voluntary sector, users, carers and supporters

- The information and social histories gathered following admission should always consider the views of other family members, carers and persons close to the patient. Their views should also be sought when Care Programme Approach plans are made before discharge and when they are reviewed after discharge. The only exception should be when the patient has made a formal declaration of unwillingness for them to be involved. Key workers should receive training in the most effective ways of establishing these communicating links and of managing the sometimes delicate ethical issues involved in maintaining them. This process should be incorporated in the checklist of subjects discussed with their work supervisors *(Sinclair p.76).*

- The clinical team should inform the patient's nearest relative of their right to request an assessment themselves where the carer believes that the patient should be in hospital and the patient is refusing any admission offered *(Hampshire p.72)*.

- Relatives must be made aware that they have free access to the clinical team and should be encouraged to contact them with any concerns about the patient or his/her carer *(Hampshire p.72)*.

- The implementation of the existing multi-agency initiatives in relation to carer support should be given high priority *(Viner p.52)*.

- Steps should be taken to incorporate current guidance into local practice and procedure including the following:
  - carers should be involved in planning care;
  - care plans should be agreed with carers as far as possible;
  - carers may need their own needs assessed *(Viner p.53)*.

- Any assessment under the Care Programme Approach should include a full appraisal of the situation and potential difficulties of the carer - especially when that person is elderly and the burden of caring is unshared *(Viner p.70)*.

- Health authorities which have no alternative but to commission the placement of patients long distances from their homes should make available funds to enable relatives and close friends to visit patients where this is beneficial to their care and rehabilitation *(Woodley p.51)*.

- Kneesworth House Hospital should develop and implement a strategy which ensures that the clinical teams place more emphasis on therapeutic intervention with patients, including recognition of the need to empower patients by training and providing information about signs and symptoms patients can recognise in themselves *(Woodley p.52)*.

- Kneesworth House Hospital should develop and implement a policy for involving patient advocates. Although we are pleased about revisions that have been made to their complaints procedure, we believe there is still a need for independent advocacy *(Woodley p.52)*.

- Committees of charitable organisations should be, and should be seen to be, independent of their employed officers and staff. New members of the committee and the committee chairman should be selected by existing committee members. It should be recognised that committee membership confers management responsibilities. There should be regular communication between committee members and senior members of staff as well as the chief officer. Members of the committee have a statutory obligation to visit the organisation and a moral obligation to spend time there and get to know staff and residents *(Newby p.154)*.

- Committees should never let one person become their sole source of information about the state of affairs in the charity's work. There should always be regular personal contact between a number of committee members (not just the chair) and a number of senior staff, in an organisation of any size. No other approach is as effective as such personal contacts *(Newby p.154)*.

- Management information should be required on all the main aspects of the charity's work. In the case of the Cyrenians, housing management, care services, staffing matters and complaints should have been monitored along with developments and finance. Committees should not be deterred from questioning either the figures presented or why other information has not been presented *(Newby p.155)*.

- Committee representatives should be involved in the recruitment of the next tier of managers below the chief officer. Such posts should be openly advertised *(Newby p.155)*.

- Committee members should regularly and actively monitor the quality of services actually being provided, either seeing it themselves first hand or obtaining independent reports *(Newby p.155)*.

- Employees should be able to make direct representations to committee officers or members where line management fails to communicate legitimate complaints regarding the care of clients and the management of services. The Nolan Committee's suggestion that public bodies should designate an official or board member to investigate staff concerns may well be equally relevant to the charity sector *(Newby p.155)*.

- The Trust should consider inviting relatives or friends to the initial appointment and to subsequent reviews so that a fuller picture of the patient's background can be obtained *(Boland p.29)*.

- More time should be set aside for discussions with relatives about care and treatment plans, and they should be welcomed at case conferences.... The key task in working with relatives is to engage them in the overall care plan so that they become partners with the clinical team in their relative's care. ... Professionals need to be trained to trust the experienced judgement of close family, rather than rely on their own impressions made at one isolated assessment *(The Falling Shadow p.147)*.

- Trust should formulate a clear statement of intent about their approach to the involvement of service users and relatives in the development and management of services for people with learning disabilities *(Thameside p.26)*.

- There should be local development of:
  - ▲ Code of Practice for User Involvement and Empowerment; and
  - ▲ Good Practice Standards on Working with Carers
  - ▲ regular 'Consumer Surveys' seeking the views of recent users about the quality of care they had received *(S.Devon p.86)*.

- The mental health service should have its own designated complaints officer to develop a special expertise in investigating complaints of mentally disordered patients. One possibility is an advocacy scheme to assist users in expressing their views *(S.Devon p.87)*.

- Support for the setting up of a local Mental Health User Group Co-Ordinator *(S.Devon p.87)*.

- Clear guidelines should be produced concerning basic information which should be available to home owners/carers *(Usoro p.17)*.

- Immediate establishment of an adequately resources patients advocacy service, independently constituted and managed, with completely trained personnel *(Ashworth p.257)*.

- Families and informal carers of patients need to be more fully informed about treatment and more closely involved in care planning for patients if they wish. Consultants should be encouraged to see the families of mental health in-patients and to use relatives' knowledge of patients *(Oxfordshire p.9)*.

- Means should be found to ensure that voluntary service activities in mental health are continued ... since such activities are vital to the effective operation of the "Care in the Community" policy *(N.Lincolnshire p.x)*.

- The efforts being made ... to secure improved and extended "drop-in" facilities should receive sympathetic consideration and support by the statutory agencies *(N.Lincolnshire p.x).*

- The contribution of the voluntary sector should be recognised and developed within the Partnership Group *(N.Lincolnshire p.x).*

PSYCHIATRIC SERVICES - Day Care / employment

- The Chief Executive of the Trust ensures that the issue of consultant responsibility of the Day Hospital is resolved without delay *(Gadher p.30).*

- All referrals to the Star Centre of patients subject to the Care Programme Approach procedure should be accompanied by full Care Programme Approach documentation *(Gadher p.33).*

- All referrals to the Heston Work Centre or to any other day care resource of patients subject to the Care Programme Approach procedure should be accompanied by full Care Programme Approach documentation *(Gadher p.34).*

- Large institutional day centres should be reprovided in local areas *(Woodley p.107).*

- The assessment of an individual's day care needs should form part of comprehensive assessment (through the care programme approach or care management, and individual care plans devised which tailor services to the needs of individuals. In consequence, the traditional method of referral by day centre application form should be reviewed *(Woodley p.107).*

- Where the primary benefit to some service users who have a serious and enduring mental illness of using day centre facilities, has been to develop self confidence and social skills, consideration should be given to promoting user empowerment by encouraging self-management arrangements with a lower staffing complement, in premises which reflect ordinary life principles (e.g. community centres), and in smaller groups which reflect common interests *(Woodley p.107).*

- In community care assessments and reviews, greater prominence be given to issues of access and personal support needs of people wishing to re-enter open employment *(Woodley p.107).*

- Where the primary benefit of day services to some service users is rehabilitative or therapeutic, the skills and experiences of day care support workers should be tailored towards meeting individual rather than group needs, with outreach to enable social integration in the community *(Woodley p.108).*

- The Trust should clarify the roles and responsibilities of the junior doctors, the Consultant and the Senior Registrar, in relation to the Day Hospital. The clarification should be incorporated in the operational policy of the Day Hospital *(Boland p.29).*

- The Trust must ensure that a policy is established and procedures written down so that the Care Programme Approach is implemented in respect of discharges from the Day Hospital, as well as from inpatient care *(Boland p.30).*

SOCIAL SERVICES DEPARTMENTS - General

- All referrals to the social services department should be in writing (this excludes referrals directly to the attached Community Mental Health Team social worker) *(Viner p.65)*.

- If a referral is made to a social worker within a Community Mental Health Team then that person must have access to original referral documents and details of any subsequent assessments undertaken *(Viner p.65)*.

- If the social services department is asked to become involved in a specific piece of work by health professionals, the existing care plan must be made available, evaluated and understood *(Viner p.65)*.

- Robust attempts should be made to retrieve any existing family or personal history from social services records to facilitate assessment and diagnosis of persons admitted to hospital secure units, and with a view to future social work involvement *(Woodley p.52)*.

- Departments of Social Services have both statutory and moral responsibilities to those requiring community care for mental illness who are receiving services from voluntary organisations. Terms of contracts with these organisations should be defined so that standards relate to those of statutory health and social services and the standards should be reviewed systematically on a case review basis. Means of access to the advice and experience of Approved Social Workers should be defined and availability made public for the benefit of clients' carers and agencies providing care *(Newby p.151)*.

- The Social Services Department should review their procedures for recording information about people with whom they have been involved. While there is in existence a system for recording assessments and on-going contacts, there seems to be no adequate retrieval system for recording requests for information by outside organisations or for recording how such requests are relayed or actioned *(Boland p.31)*.

- When the planning of organisational change is underway, attention should be given to a detailed and critical analysis of the effects of change likely to occur at the interface between the 'old' and the 'new' with particular regard for the needs of children on the child protection register. Additional resources, directed to ensure a smooth handover in such cases are necessary, e.g. an increase in front line staff for the transition period *(Dalson p.12)*.

- More social workers should be recruited where teams are seen to be under strength in particular if the team is involved with new referrals *(Clunis p.120)*.

- Where social services reception and referral systems are manned by unqualified or inexperienced staff, such staff must have ready access to an experienced Approved Social Worker *(Clunis p.120)*.

- Unqualified and recently qualified social workers must work under the supervision of a qualified and experienced manager and their work should be reviewed at least once every fortnight by their supervisors *(Clunis p.120)*.

- When current cases involve active danger the daily hand over and briefing arrangements for staff should ensure that the case continues to receive prompt attention *(Clunis p.120)*.

- There should be close contact and liaison between social services departments and local housing agencies *(Clunis p.120).*

- A hospital social worker attending ward rounds/case conferences should make the Social Services Department aware of the individual's existence in all cases *(Rooney p.34).*

- A clearer policy and procedure for referral of patients to Social Services should be introduced *(N.Lincolnshire p.xii).*

- Better communication arrangements should be introduced to ensure that social work support is available to all patients, regardless of source of referral *(N.Lincolnshire p.xiii).*

- Medical and nursing staff in particular should be encouraged to give full consideration to use of the support available from the Social Services Department *(N.Lincolnshire p.xiii).*

- Full and developing use should be made of Social Services facilities (such as hostel places and places in Part III accommodation) *(N.Lincolnshire p.xiii).*

- Supervision should be planned on the basis that the choice of cases for discussion should be that of the supervisor, while, of course, giving the social worker being supervised the opportunity to discuss cases where s/he wants help and advice. The supervisor will need to have a system to ensure that all cases are covered periodically. If there is a requirement for the supervisor to sign the notes read at supervision, the signature should appear at the end of the last note, so that, when next reviewed, the supervisor can readily see what entries have been made since last read *(Campbell p.74).*

- Local Authorities should provide guidelines on supervision which should, in general terms, indicate the scope and purposes of supervision (including scrutiny of records), the interval at which supervision should occur (varying according to the experience and seniority of the social worker) and the approximate maximum interval that should elapse between consideration of cases held by a social worker *(Campbell p.75).*

- Social Workers should be given guidance on the ways to recognise and if possible avert incidents of violence and that the employing authorities should make written guidelines available. Social Workers should report incidents of violence and threatened violence and counselling should be available to social workers *(Campbell p.75).*

- Personal audible alarms should be made available to social workers and support staff if they wish to have them *(Campbell p.76).*

- Departments should appoint a named individual with responsibility for oversight of the office security arrangements and for periodic testing of alarms and security systems *(Campbell p.76).*

SOCIAL SERVICES DEPARTMENTS - Approved Social Workers

- Social Services Departments which transfer case responsibility for restricted patients should also transfer the case records *(Mitchell p.46).*

- Any social services worker assigned the task of social supervisor of a restricted patient should be an Approved Social Worker *(Mitchell p.240)*.

- Copies of any notes/report made by an Approved Social Worker for an assessment prior to an application for a s.2 Order should be made available to the hospital within 3 days and read at the earliest opportunity by the RMO or his Junior Doctor and the Named Nurse responsible for the patient and kept on the patient's file(s) *(Grey p.49)*.

- An Approved Social Worker should be available in each social services department to respond to crises and to provide advice. An Approved Social Worker should be contactable throughout the working day, as well as at night and during weekends and public holidays *(Clunis p.120)*.

- Medical recommendations leading to detention should be copied for the Approved Social Worker for his records, and a copy of the Application for Admission recommendation should be kept by him. He should also provide a report for the Hospital where the patient is to be detained and retain a copy of it for the social services file on the patient *(Clunis p.120)*.

- ASW failed to comply with s.11(3), Mental Health Act 1983 and inform the Nearest Relative of the application for admission to hospital and of their power of discharge *(Barratt p.7)*.

GENERAL PRACTITIONERS

- The GP for any patient subject to the Care Programme Approach should be provided with a copy of any care plan and informed of any change to that plan *(Viner p.23)*.

- Where a person cared for is subject to the Care Programme Approach then, subject to consent (and taking into account the needs of confidentiality) the keyworker ought to ensure that the carer's GP is provided with a copy of the care plan *(Viner p.24)*.

- There should be formal arrangement for routine joint review of all the GP practice clients who are in receipt of care from the specialist mental health team. This would allow cases to be discussed and reviewed at practice meetings attended by Community Psychiatric Nurses *(Viner p.24)*.

- The care plan must specify who has medical responsibility. Where the GP has the responsibility s/he must be involved in all significant decisions affecting medical care. In such cases the opinion of the consultant psychiatrist can only be advisory *(Southampton p.10)*.

- GP participation in care planning should be sought wherever possible *(Southampton p.10)*.

- The prescribing practices of GP's for depression should be the subject of clinical audit leading to the establishment of protocols *(Southampton p.10)*.

- The role of primary care prescribing in the treatment of complex mental health cases needs to be reviewed jointly between primary care and the specialist services *(Southampton p.10)*.

- We think there may be value in further discussions at a national level between police and GP representatives in order to address the issue of collaboration in respect of crisis situations involving people with mental illness who are potentially violent. Arrangements also require to be agreed in local areas between GP's, psychiatric services, mental health officers and the police with reference to collaborating over such emergency situations *(McFadden - Scotland p.27)*.

- As a general issue, the development of community care requires that the training of the police be appraised to ensure that there is adequate preparation for recognising mental illness and dealing with members of the public who are mentally ill *(McFadden - Scotland p.27)*.

- Before a GP may remove a patient from his list, whom he believes or suspects suffers from a psychiatric illness, he must obtain advice from the local Psychiatric team and follow such advice, and must inform the Family Health Services Authority of his intention to remove the patient from his list, so that the Authority can ensure that the patient is registered with a new GP as soon as possible *(Clunis p.128)*.

- A GP whose patient is on the Supervision Register or aftercare under s.117, Mental Health Act 1983 must not remove the patient from their list without previously informing the patient's Responsible Medical Officer, and ensuring that another GP has agreed to act as the patient's GP *(Clunis p.128)*.

- The Royal College of Psychiatrists should be asked to design a crisis card for mentally ill people. GP's should encourage the use of the card *(Clunis p.128)*.

- GP's should familiarise themselves with the patient's previous mental, as well as medical, history *(Usoro p.17)*.

- The GP must be clear where s/he fits into the community care plan, whether he will be simply a point of contact in an emergency, whom s/he should contact at the community psychiatric service, or whether the patient's mental illness will be completely managed by community psychiatric staff *(Usoro p.17)*.

- If the GP does provide an initial emergency service or makes any substantial change to the treatment programme including medication, s/he must report such actions to the key worker at the earliest opportunity *(Usoro p.17)*.

- GP's should not prescribe psychotropic medication by telephone without first reviewing the patient *(Usoro p.17)*.

- A general practice has round the clock responsibility to the practice patients. This responsibility includes provision when the practice doctors are off duty. When all members of a practice are off duty, it is the doctors' responsibility to ensure that an efficient deputising service is available and functioning *(Usoro p.17)*.

- There should be prompt information available to GP's concerning any significant change in patient circumstances. New GP's who are awaiting transfer of medical records should receive basic information about the patient from the Care Manager as soon as ever practicable (Usoro p.17).

- GP's should routinely be informed of the following:-
  - a patient has been admitted;
  - a patient has gone absent without leave;
  - a patient has been discharged; and
  - details of any medication or treatment regime including what (if any) medication he is believed to have in his possession *(Rooney pp.25/26)*.

- Also if patients fail to attend out-patient appointments *(Rooney pp.36, 38)*.

COMMUNITY PSYCHIATRIC NURSES

- Where a Community Psychiatric Nurse is sent in by the treating doctors to assess the patient who they believe should be in hospital i.e. to be the eyes and ears of the clinical team, a detailed record of what is seen and heard at each visit must be sent to the doctors as soon as possible with copies to the GP *(Hampshire p.72)*.

- No Community Psychiatric Nurse with primary responsibility for a patient should go on leave without making cover arrangements for high priority patients and without notifying the patient's GP *(Hampshire p.72)*.

- The Trust and the Health Authority should review the provision of community psychiatric nurses and address any underresourcing *(Boland p.30)*.

- The Trust should work with the purchasing authorities to ensure that there is no contractual disincentive to discharge patients from Community Psychiatric Nurse caseloads whilst they remain ill and a danger to themselves or others *(Buchanan p.23)*.

- The caseloads of Community Psychiatric Nurses should be reviewed to ensure that they reflect a reasonable level of workload. Community Psychiatric Nurse caseloads should be reported to management at regular intervals for monitoring purposes *(Buchanan p.23)*.

- Guidelines should be produced for Community Psychiatric Nurses explaining the circumstances when a patient who declines a service or goes missing can be discharged from their caseloads *(Buchanan p.23)*.

- Community Psychiatric Nurses should not be able to discharge former inpatients from caseloads without gaining the prior agreement of the responsible medical officer or nurse manager *(Buchanan p.23)*.

- For patients known to be a risk to themselves or others, or likely to break down in the community, a policy should be developed for dealing with them should they fail to maintain contact with their Community Psychiatric Nurse *(Buchanan p.23)*.

- The management of the Mental Health Unit should explore ways in which the appropriate community psychiatric nurse can be informed at an early date about a patient in hospital when it is likely that the community psychiatric nurse will subsequently be involved in that patient's care. The community psychiatric nurse should then be involved, wherever practicable, in making the arrangements for the patient's discharge *(Findlay p.18)*.

- A clear decision should be reached as to the appropriate caseload for Community Psychiatric Nurses, in line with regional or national guidelines, and the number of Community Psychiatric Nurses should be increased with a view to reducing their caseloads accordingly *(Simpson p.108)*.

    a) Consideration should be given, in discussion with GP's and other appropriate interests, to the establishment of arrangements whereby depot injections may be given by GP practice nurses or by Community Psychiatric Nurses at health clinics rather than by individual visits on the part of Community Psychiatric Nurses.

b) Consideration should be given to establishing the nursing process within the Community Psychiatric Nurse service in a form as close as practicable to that used within the hospital and to the provision of appropriate training thereon.
c) Management should ensure that Community Psychiatric Nurses have appropriate training and experience. *(Simpson p 108).*

- Improved induction and supervision arrangements for Community Psychiatric Nurses should be introduced, in particular for those staff working in isolated situations *(N.Lincolnshire p.xi).*

- Where the decision to discontinue treating a patient in the community is taken by a Community Psychiatric Nurse, this should be clearly communicated both to the patient's GP and also (where appropriate) to the Consultant *(N.Lincolnshire p.xii).*

CHILDREN

- Local social services and health authorities should address the support needs of parents with severe mental health problems, and the needs of their children, in community care plans and in children's services plans, and allocate resources. In so doing, that they review the distribution, co-ordination and access to specialist mental health services for children and families *(Woodley p.21).*

- Area Child Protection Committees should raise awareness of mental health issues and promote good inter-agency practices *(Woodley p.21).*

- Where children assume the role of carer in households with a mentally ill parent, the principles expounded in the small study by Leeds SSD (p.20 - Woodley Team Report) should be adopted by health, education and social services authorities *(Woodley p.21).*

- Strategies which aim to improve attendance at child protection conferences should continue to be developed, monitored and regularly reviewed. It was noted that different Area Offices programmed conferences on specific days to give good prior notice to invitees in order to reduce delays and improve attendance. More recently a conference report form had been devised requesting completing by invitees if they ware unable to attend *(Dalson p.13).*

- Consideration should be given to the provision of a handwritten decision sheet prepared at the conference and outlining family composition, those present, decisions and recommendations and date of next meeting. This would be taken away with participants and distributed to absentees without delay thus assisting the speedy dissemination of information from conferences to all relevant personnel *(Dalson p.13).*

- Adult psychiatrists may be unfamiliar with child protection issues. Guidance on the communication expectations for the psychiatric services when they are treating a patent where there are child protection issues should be formulated *(Dalson p.13).*

- In cases where there is an alleged criminal aspect professionals should read the police statements which give a first hand account of incidents in which the client has been involved *(Dalson p.13).*

- The Chair should routinely ask for the children's views on the situation under discussion and be informed of the efforts made to gain their views *(Dalson p.13).*

- More attention should be given to listening and talking with children. Working directly with children should be essential training for social workers involved with children and their families *(Dalson p.14).*

- There should be a standard item on all child protection conference agendas to consider issues of race and culture *(Dalson p.14).*

- It should become Social Services procedure that Minority Ethnic Liaison Officers must be formally consulted on all child protection cases where issues of race and culture have been identified as having an impact on effective intervention in a family *(Dalson p.14).*

- In cases where legal action may be required the Chair should ensure that the team manager and social worker involved in the case discuss legal options with a lawyer from the local authority legal section *(Dalson p.14).*

- A system should be set up to monitor that child protection review conferences are held at the required intervals as specified in the child protection procedures *(Dalson p.15).*

- There should be a requirement that specific child protection training be undertaken by newly qualified social workers before they assume responsibility for child protection cases *(Dalson p.15).*

- Transfer summaries on child protection cases should provide an overview of the case and be explicit about the work with the family that must proceed without disruption. Negotiation regarding handover arrangements between outgoing and incoming team managers must take place in order to ensure that the primary goal of maintaining adequate protection of the children continues to be met *(Dalson p.15).*

THE ASSESSMENT AND MANAGEMENT OF RISK

- Directors of Mental Health Services and Directors of Social Services should ensure that all professional staff who work with psychiatric patients become familiar, and remain familiar, with the indicators of dangerousness and are confident of what action to take should they encounter them *(Sinclair p.77).*

- Managers of the appropriate agencies should ensure that all staff who are involved in the implementation of the Care Programme Approach are trained in risk assessment *(Armstrong p.100).*

- The clinicians have a clear responsibility to seek the views of the immediate family in a situation where the medical opinion is that the patient should be in hospital and the patient refuses informal admission. The family should be involved if possible in the taking of any history and in the assessment of the patient's current condition especially when the patient is being cared for in the community and is refusing or unable to attend outpatient appointments. A proper risk assessment should always include the views of the family where possible *(Hampshire p.71).*

- If the treating doctor examines the patient and is of the opinion that the patient needs hospitalisation, is not at that time sectionable and is refusing to be admitted informally, there must be a continuous process of risk assessment which must include regular face to face review by the clinicians. Part of that assessment must include the health and safety of any carer. Clinicians should be encouraged to try to identify patterns in the patient's mood and behaviour. An assessment must not be made over the telephone *(Hampshire p.72)*.

- As part of the risk assessment which must be carried out by the clinical team, consideration should be given to referral to an Approved Social Worker to carry out an assessment *(Hampshire p.72)*.

- Risk assessment should be an integral part of the Care Programme Approach documentation circulated *(Gadher p.32)*.

- Risk assessment training should be extended to all Community Mental Health Team members *(Viner p.70)*.

- A multidisciplinary panel with representatives from all the relevant mental health, mental handicap, social work, probation and education services, should be established to consider the most appropriate care package for at risk patients where there is uncertainty as to which agency should be the one to take the lead caring role. An appropriate chairperson for such a panel would be a forensic psychiatrist. The main role of this panel would be to resolve inter-agency disputes and uncertainties about the "ownership" of people who did not fit into the standard services on offer *(Doherty - N.Ireland p.79)*.

- The Mental Health Services and other relevant disciplines in the Western Board area should co-operate to identify patients using defined criteria for at risk patients for inclusion in the supervision group. A specialist team led by a forensic psychiatrist with access to back up medium secure unit beds should be established. The specialist team should be multidisciplinary in nature *(Doherty - N.Ireland p.81)*.

- Local social services and district health authorities review their policies and procedures for risk assessment and risk management, in conjunction with service users, for the following purposes:
  - internal transmission of confidential personal information between service units on a 'need to know' basis;
  - disclosure to external agencies providing community care services on a 'need to know' basis;
  - production of a service user consent form;
  - inclusion in Health and Safety at Work and 'Violence' Guidelines *(Woodley p.108)*.

- Without all available information, accurate risk assessment becomes impossible. We would, therefore, urge that an index of essential documentation is developed to serve as a check list for newly-referred patients. This should form the basis of a minimum documentation standard, at least in relation to patients with a forensic background, or on supervision (or mental health priority) registers *(The Falling Shadow p.140)*.

- When a patient is referred for the first time, or transferred from another ream, there should always be a new clinical assessment which should include an assessment of risk of violence *(The Falling Shadow p.177)*.

- Development of a risk management strategy aimed at promoting the safety and security of patients, staff and the public. The strategy must contain:-
  - mechanisms for informing staff of individual patient's propensities to violence;
  - assessment of the environment, including community locations;
  - an incident reporting system, and review system;
  - a continuing programme of staff training *(S.Devon pp.52, 84)*.

- The Consultant Psychiatrist with responsibility for the patient must assess, together with the multi-disciplinary team, the risk of the patient harming himself or others *(Clunis p.110)*.

- All members of the team should be alerted to signs and symptoms in the patient which may indicate that the patient is likely to relapse. Such signs and symptoms may be identified by the doctors but may also be identified by the patient himself or his relatives or friends. Non compliance with medication should be recognised as a significant pointer to a relapse *(Clunis p.110)*.

- An accurate record should be made of any incident of violence and the details should be included in the patient's discharge summary *(Clunis p.119)*.

- An assessment of the risk of dangerousness should be included in the discharge summary whenever the patient has acted with violence *(Clunis p.119)*.

- Everyone who has contact in their professional or service work with mentally ill people who may pose a risk of violence should have training in the assessment of dangerousness, and understand when to refer the patient for expert guidance *(Clunis p.119)*.

- Need for training on risk assessment *(Rooney pp.36,38)*.

- Any record of violence or potential violence, including medical and nursing or social work notes, should follow a patient on transfer and be made available to all staff newly concerned with that patient's care *(Inweh p.4)*.

- Any incidents of violence or potential violence should be fully discussed at predischarge meetings and at the Accommodation Panel if hostel or residential care within the community is being considered *(Inweh p.6)*.

- While we accept there is a reluctance to apply pejorative labels to patients we recommend that where serious violence has occurred, full reports should be made available to all those who need to know *(Inweh p.6)*.

- Kingston MIND should draw up a policy in respect of violence at work and offer training to its staff in the prevention, early recognition and management of violence *(Inweh p.7)*.

- In all cases where violence, or potential violence has been a factor, a full consideration before discharge should take place on any history of previous incidents, and this should be available to all the professionals and agencies involved *(Inweh p.9)*.

- Clinical teams should seek to use the best available actuarial, statistical or predictive techniques to support clinical judgements about dangerousness *(Kirkman p.35)*.

- Clinical teams should increasingly develop the use of neurophysiological, and psychometric tests to support clinical judgements about dangerousness *(Kirkman p.35)*.

- All who provide services for mentally disordered offenders should strongly encourage or commission research into the improved classification of personality disorder and methods of predicting dangerousness *(Kirkman p.37)*.

- Although it is recognised that the evaluation whilst in hospital of a patient's dangerousness is very difficult, full weight should be given during that evaluation not only to the patient's current behaviour but also to any previous events *(Findlay p.18)*.

- Where a patient in a psychiatric hospital is found in possession of a knife or similar weapon, in circumstances where its possession is unauthorised or concealed, a record should be made in the patient's notes of the circumstances and any subsequent action *(Campbell p.74)*.

POLICE SERVICE

- All Police Forces should have formal Missing Patients Procedures agreed with local hospitals and Social Services, and within these a system for inquiring into the circumstances of repeated absconding by detained patients, particularly those subject to restriction orders *(Mitchell p.205)*.

- Police Forces nation-wide should commit themselves to adopting the training and policies for dealing with mentally ill people, as currently practised within the Metropolitan Police *(Mitchell p.238)*.

- The police are asked to review their procedures for notifying the specialist agencies in the case of any concerns they may have about individual clients *(Southampton p.11)*.

- The police should when considering the need for medical treatment under custody procedures, include consideration of the need for psychiatric treatment in the case of prisoners believed to be experiencing mental ill health *(Woodley p.130)*.

- When a person taken into police custody for a serious crime can reasonably be suspected of significant recent use of alcohol or non-prescribed drugs a police surgeon should be summoned rapidly so that appropriate testing can be carried out, subject to the consent of the suspect *(Newby p.153)*.

- The police should keep a log of all telephone calls which have been "cut off" accidentally or deliberately *(Newby p.153)*.

- The police should ensure that police switchboard operators inform the radio operator of all calls which have been deliberately terminated *(Newby p.153)*.

- Procedures and documentation re. s.136, Mental Health Act 1983 should be standardised *(Clunis p.127)*.

- Officers should be given proper training in mental illness. It is vital that such training should include both knowledge about mental illness and experience of those who suffer from mental illness *(Clunis p.127)*.

- The Police should be encouraged to liaise with local community mental health services *(Clunis p.127)*.

- An officer should be appointed at every Police Station to deal with mental health issues *(Clunis p.127)*.

- Expectation that the Police would establish whether person was an absconder or wanted for any offence elsewhere as a matter of routine and should be prepared to pass this information to doctors along with any information which may help determine whether he is at risk (e.g. offences of violence or where he has in the past been committed to a hospital, perhaps in another part of the country) *(Rooney p.39)*.

- In those cases where the police have preferred or are considering preferring charges on a hospital patient they should supply a written note to the hospital management requesting to be informed when the patient is about to leave hospital. The note should indicate the seriousness of the charge and the alleged facts where these involve any danger to life or limb. In the event of the police subsequently deciding not to prefer charges a further written notification should be sent to the hospital *(Findlay p.17)*.

- In a case where the police have requested information on the movements of a patient it is the hospital management's responsibility to form a judgement between the public interest and the confidentiality of its relationship with the patient. If a decision to disclose information is made any notification to the police about the actual or imminent discharge of a patient should be made, or confirmed, in writing *(Findlay p.17)*.

MENTALLY DISORDERED OFFENDERS

- In any case where the criminal event involving a mentally disordered person is serious or dangerous, it should be the responsibility of the Crown Prosecution Service to prepare a full account of the criminal event before criminal proceedings have been finalised. The CPS should also ensure that this account is transmitted, after the criminal process has run its course, to all those involved in the criminal proceedings, to clinicians subsequently responsible for the care of the patient, and to C3 Division of the Home Office in respect of restricted cases. The account should become an established part of the patient's clinical record *(Mitchell p.120)*.

- The Crown Prosecution Service should review its procedures in relation to the prosecution of mentally disordered offenders destined to be routed into the mental health system through a Hospital Order *(Mitchell p.121)*.

- The Royal College of Psychiatrists, the Royal College of Nursing and other relevant professional bodies, should issue guidance to their respective members not to rest content with information about the 'index offence' but to inquire thoroughly into the criminal events *(Mitchell p.125)*.

- In-patient units whose patients include offenders with disturbed personalities should have access to specialist psychodynamic expertise *(Mitchell p.170)*.

- RMO's and clinicians managing offender patients should afford such patients regular interviews in private *(Mitchell p.177)*.

- All trainees in General Psychiatry should spend a period of training in a forensic psychiatric service under the supervision of a Forensic Psychiatrist *(Mitchell p.244)*.

- General Psychiatrists taking up consultant posts with responsibility for secure beds should have had a period of training in forensic psychiatry *(Mitchell p.244).*

- Arrangements for psychiatric training both nationally and locally in Suffolk and in the Anglia and Oxford Region, should be reviewed and, if necessary, enhanced so as to ensure that all trainees in general psychiatry receive adequate clinical training, and experience in psychodynamic and forensic aspects of psychiatry *(Mitchell p.245).*

- Health service providers with responsibility for mental health service users who have a forensic history should ensure there is a jointly produced protocol and criteria concerning follow up arrangements by forensic and general consultant psychiatrists, applicable to the area of residence of the service user and in consultation with local social services authorities *(Woodley p.108).*

- The interface between forensic and general mental health service provision be reviewed *(Woodley p.110).*

- The Trust should establish guidelines for offering assistance to the police or Prison Service when a known patient is held in custody. These will need to address the issue of when and in what circumstances the professional duty of patient confidentiality should be overridden *(Boland p.30).*

- Provision of guidance to health authorities and mental health providers on the appropriate use of s.37, Mental Health Act 1983 and its value in providing medium term treatment for people with personality disorders, especially those who have a 'treatable' mental illness component to their disorder *(Buchanan p.24).*

- A system for assessing mentally ill offenders over a long term period taking account of their criminal records and mental state assessments. Where a pattern of repeated episodes of criminal activity linked to mental illness is apparent, assessment for detention under an enhanced hospital order should be undertaken *(Buchanan p.25).*

- There is a clear need for an increased number of forensic psychiatrists *(Clunis p.123).*

- Every psychiatric service should include a doctor who has a special interest in Forensic Psychiatry *(Clunis p.123).*

- A medical recommendation obtained by the Police in relation to a mentally disordered offender, must be sent to the Crown Prosecution Service with the papers or as soon as possible thereafter as it is received *(Clunis p.126).*

- The Consultant Psychiatrist who is responsible for the care of a patient, who has been charged with an offence and remanded to hospital, must consider whether the patient needs to be detained for treatment under the Mental Health Act 1983, irrespective of the outcome of that charge *(Clunis p.126).*

- The Forensic Psychiatric Services and the local Police Forces should jointly devise a liaison policy to guide procedure in the investigation of patients who are suspected of serious personal crime. The policy should include a description of what remedies or disciplinary action might be taken where individuals deviate from agreed guidance. Regional Health Authorities should keep a check on these *(Kirkman pp.36, 38).*

- Psychiatrists should provide Magistrates, safeguarding confidentiality, with information about their patients who have been arrested and who have a history of mentally abnormal offending, to enable the most appropriate remand to be made *(Kirkman p.36).*

PROBATION SERVICE

- Statutory involvement of the Probation Service with mentally disordered offenders should be at the discretion of the courts where there is a need for such contact rather than being dependent on the sentences given *(Buchanan p.25).*

- Representatives of the District Health Authority and the Probation Service should meet periodically in a formal context to monitor and encourage co-operation in working relationships *(N.Lincolnshire p.x).*

PRISON SERVICE

- The Prison Service should ensure, by the end of 1996, that it has in place a database and a fully effective system whereby prisoners' Inmate Medical Records, including those of remand prisoners, follow them wherever they may be in the system. The provision should encompass access to the system for all those involved in the penal system *(Mitchell p.262).*

- The question of confidentiality of prison medical records should be fully reviewed. As a first step towards such review, the General Medical Council and other professional bodies should be asked for their views *(Mitchell p.267).*

- There should be far greater liaison between prison and hospital upon transfer of patients under section. A written summary of any relevant observed behaviour in the prison (including if possible a copy of any Incident Report form in relation to the prisoner) should be sent to the hospital at the time of transfer. At the very least there should be telephone contact between the Principal Officer on the relevant prison wing and the Charge Nurse on the receiving ward at the hospital to discuss any significant behavioural problems *(Grey p.49).*

- The Prison medical/nursing notes including copies of the section transfer documents should go straight to the patient's hospital file and remain there until discharge, when they should be photocopied and returned to the prison *(Grey p.49).*

- The Trust should, at the earliest opportunity, set up a meeting with Pentonville Prison medical service, the probation and social services, to discuss the concerns and recommendations outlined in this report. They should further agree an action plan for their implementation and to improve communication and cooperation between their separate agencies *(Grey p.51).*

- The prison service should have guidelines for the health care staff about the care of mentally disordered people in prison, particularly with regard to seeking an opinion from the catchment area psychiatrist, rather than transferring inmates from prison to prison, keeping people in minimally furnished cells, or persistently medicating them against their will *(Woodley p.33).*

- The prison service should implements a better administrative procedure for keeping its health care records (as we believe very useful information could be lost with the present system, which has resulted in vital records being misplaced and not traceable: computerisation could be a solution) *(Woodley p.33)*.

- Patients with a mental illness detained in prison should have the right to regular consultation with a qualified psychiatrist *(Buchanan p.25)*.

- Prison Medical Officers should receive training in the psychiatric treatment of mentally ill offenders and be involved in their discharge planning *(Buchanan p.25)*.

IN-PATIENT CARE - General

- Nurses must ensure that a comprehensive history is taken on admission and updated regularly and in our view the Roper - Logan - Tierney model is not suitable for the recording of this information in Psychiatry *(Armstrong p.97)*.

- There must be adequate supervision of the history taking exercise and recording of information when it is undertaken by a student nurse *(Armstrong p.97)*.

- The opportunity must exist for the medical and nursing history to be amplified by a social work history when considered appropriate *(Armstrong p.98)*.

- The role and responsibilities of nursing staff at all levels should be clarified in order to facilitate improved communication *(Armstrong p.98)*.

- Patients admitted to the Acute Unit with episodes of self harm should be automatically notified to the In-Patient Psychiatric Unit, the RMO (if applicable) and to the GP *(Armstrong p.99)*.

- External Agencies (i.e. the Police, Social Services etc.) should communicate with the RMO when they are investigating an In-Patient who is known to be under the RMO's care *(Armstrong p.99)*.

- The patient should not be allocated to a Named Nurse who is on leave or off sick at the time of admission to hospital or transfer from one ward to another *(Grey p.49)*.

- All doctors who undertake the role of RMO on a permanent or temporary basis should be informed of their full range of responsibilities and duties, and those which can and cannot be delegated *(Grey p.49)*.

- The medical and nursing notes should be kept if possible in the same file or at least in the same place so that there is ready access to all relevant information *(Grey p.49)*.

- All relevant information about a patient (such as the name of his RMO, the section of the MHA he is detained under and the date of any removal of the section, the fact that he is AWOL and the date of discharge from the hospital) should be logged onto the hospital computer as soon as possible after such detail comes into existence and should be updated with any change *(Grey p.49)*.

- All new inpatients should be seen by the consultant responsible for their care or a senior psychiatrist deputising for him/her within three days of admission, unless the patient has been examined by the consultant or senior deputy at an outpatient clinic or in the community in the one/two days prior to admission *(Doherty - N.Ireland p.76)*.

- Management should arrange the consultant's contract to allow more frequent review of inpatients' progress according to the patients' needs *(Doherty - N.Ireland p.76)*.

- A detailed mental state assessment and care plan should be entered in all newly admitted patient's case notes. This should be updated at least once per week *(Doherty - N.Ireland p.77)*.

- When patients who have been detained for assessment are regraded as voluntary patients, there should be a detailed written record of the reasons for regrading *(Doherty - N.Ireland p.77)*.

- There should be an immediate review of the implementation of the named nurse procedures *(Doherty - N.Ireland p.77)*.

- The nursing staff should be reminded of their responsibilities in relation to record keeping (UKCC Standards for Records and Record Keeping, 1993) *(Doherty - N.Ireland p.77)*.

- Kneesworth House Hospital should develop and implement more positive action policies for responding to the needs of patients from ethnic minorities and the needs of women patients *(Woodley p.51)*.

- Kneesworth House Hospital should continue to develop and implement a strategy for relieving the unacceptably cramped conditions of its ward areas *(Woodley p.51)*.

- Kneesworth House Hospital should review the occupational and educational programmes available to patients in terms of their appropriateness and accessibility to the populations they serve *(Woodley p.52)*.

- Mental health units should develop a clear policy on when a personal search will be carried out. An agreement to grant leave could, for example, be made on the explicit condition that non-compliance with the terms of leave may be followed by a search, if staff have cause for concern that harmful objects may have been brought into the ward *(The Falling Shadow p.113)*.

- We think it is essential that patients, who are as much at risk of violent incidents as members of staff, should have ready access to incident alarms *(The Falling Shadow p.114)*.

- The operational policy of the ward should be reviewed to ensure that staff recognise all aspects of patient's conditions rather than addressing only the immediate and obvious signs of illness. This should embrace the broader aspects of the patient's condition over a longer term rather than responding only to clearly treatable indicators *(Buchanan p.23)*.

- The Trust should satisfy itself that there are no staff employed in the learning disabilities services with convictions that would make such employment inappropriate *(Thameside p.25)*.

- It appears that the current redevelopment of the Hackney Unit will still leave a significant shortfall in terms of bed numbers and, therefore a range of secure provisions should be developed which are closer and more accessible to the London Borough communities from which so many of the current referrals are made *(Woodley p.51)*.

- An increased number of Medium Secure Unit beds within the South East Thames RHA is urgently needed. Furthermore urgent consideration should be given as to whether an increased number of such beds should be provided for every inner city area *(Clunis p.122)*.
- There is a clear need for the provision of rehabilitation units to be available to Regional Medium Secure Units *(Clunis p.122)*.
- An increased number of beds on general psychiatric wards in London is urgently needed. Furthermore urgent consideration should be given as to whether an increased number of such beds should be provided in every inner city area *(Clunis p.122)*.
- Constant and close observation policies and procedures should include the recording of names of nurses undertaking the observation and give consideration to issues such as when patient is in the toilet or out of the ward with relatives *(NW London pp.31/32)*.
- Open wards should only be locked when staffing levels are inadequate for the clinical situation of the ward. Operational managers should insist that the detailed steps recommended in the Code of Practice are followed. Furthermore, on each occasion when a ward is locked is reported to the next Trust Board meeting, and that the Trust supply the relevant Health Authority with a quarterly tally of such events together with a brief explanation for each occasion *(NW London p.42)*.
- Development of a clear programme of refresher training to ensure that nursing skills are maintained and developed *(Blackwood p.80)*.
- Director of Nursing Services should ensure that the UKCC Code of Professional Conduct duty "to promote and safeguard the interests and well-being of the patient" is made plain to every nurse working in the hospital *(Blackwood p.81)*.
- The need to review procedure for medical review of weekend admissions *(Rooney pp.36,38)*.
- A form should be completed by the Duty Night Co-Ordinator to give to the day Senior Nurse identifying any incident and any patients who have gone absent without leave *(Rooney pp.36,38)*.
- Poor ward communication should be addressed as a matter of urgency. There should be a full handover system at each change of staff and the nurse in charge should allocate specific responsibilities to each member of staff for the duration of the shift *(Latham p.5)*.
- There should be a system for ensuring continuity of, and responsibility for, individual resident care during meal breaks, attendance at lectures etc. *(Latham p.5)*.
- Urgent consideration should be given to revising the 12 hour shift system, its effect on the residents' day and on the ability of staff to provide the highest possible standard of care throughout such a lengthy period *(Latham p.5)*.
- The Sector Managers should aim to make a daily visit to the wards. One short weekly visit to each ward is insufficient *(Latham p.7)*.

- The implementation of the IPP (Individual Performance Planning) system should receive high priority. The form should be pre-printed with headings to ensure that all areas of a person's life are addressed *(Latham p.5)*. The Sector Managers should attend the IPP meetings in their sector *(Latham p.7)*.

- A formal appraisal of the IPP process should be undertaken by Management after it has been running for one year to ensure that it is implemented consistently and effectively *(Latham p.7)*.

- Regular minuted meetings should be held at ward level to discuss general resident issues and should be attended by the appropriate Sector Manager *(Latham p.7)*.

- The Sector Managers should carry the clear responsibility for ensuring that policies are explained to, understood and implemented by the staff under their control (Latham p.7). The present method of distribution for new and amended policies should be reviewed. Staff should receive a formal presentation and, where necessary, training for each policy which applies to their area of work. Random audit should be undertaken to ensure that staff are knowledgeable about the policies which relate to their area (Latham p.9). Policies issued by the local Health Authority and those of a general nature should be kept separately from documents that need to be consulted on a daily basis *(Latham p.10)*.

- Staff should receive education to ensure that they understand the legal aspects of their work and the rights of the residents under their care *(Latham p.8)*.

- There should be a system of planned movement of trained staff to enhance innovative care practices *(Latham p.10)*.

- Each student nurse should have a named preceptor / mentor *(Latham p.10)*.

- A formal system should be introduced to enable any member of staff to refer concerns, in confidence, to the Sector Managers or the Unit General Manager *(Latham p.10)*.

- Visiting policy and procedures should help ensure maximum facilities for visiting by family and friends, and clear understanding of when visiting may be properly restricted in line with chapter 26, Mental Health Act Code of Practice *(Ashworth p.260)*.

- Applications for access to health records pre-November 1991 ought generally to be granted *(Ashworth p.261)*.

- Wards, units and hospitals need to be fully aware of each other's policies, and to discuss and co-ordinate them as far as possible. When a patient has been transferred, if the advice given by one group of carers to the next is not accepted, this should be discussed between the care teams *(Oxfordshire p.4)*.

- Ward staff need to be always on the look out for moments of critical stress for individual patients, and should implement higher levels of observation and support at such times. Policies regarding observation of patients and contract therapy should be kept under review and considered carefully in the light of each patient's needs at a particular time *(Oxfordshire p.5)*.

- In accordance with the Patient's Charter, every patient should be allocated a fully trained Key Worker, with special responsibility for co-ordinating their care. The name of the Key Worker should be recorded in the notes and be known to the patient and to the patient's relatives. Also in accordance with the Patient's Charter, all staff on wards should wear legible name badges *(Oxfordshire p.6)*.

- Managers should ensure that clinical staff, including agency nursing and locum medical staff, are fully aware of Codes of good practice, and of the policies and procedures obtaining on wards or units, and that staffing levels are sufficient to implement them. Information about Codes of Practice and ward policies and procedures should also be available to families and patients *(Oxfordshire p.6)*.

- A multi-professional review should be undertaken of special / close observation procedure and practice and implement an effective policy for the observation of patients at risk. Suitable training will be required for staff *(Shrodells p.7)*.

- The present systems for the recording of information should be reviewed and agreement over standards for the frequency of examination and recording of information about inpatients reached with medical and nursing staff. The revised standards should be submitted to the District Health Authority and subject to systematic monitoring as part of the clinical audit process *(Shrodells p.7)*.

- Present systems for the induction of staff who are new to the mental health service including agency nursing and locum medical staff should be reviewed *(Shrodells p.9)*.

- When the further detention of a patient under a section of the Mental Health Act is being considered the first stage should be a sounding out of opinions amongst staff involved in the care of the patient, together with an encouragement to express views, before a conclusion is reached. This is relevant whether the preferred option is to extend the detention or to allow it to lapse *(Findlay p.17)*.

- The lead role in a patient's nursing care should always be taken by a qualified nurse *(Findlay p.18)*.

- Entries into nursing records should normally be made by qualified staff. Where, exceptionally, entries are made by nursing assistants, they should be countersigned by a qualified nurse *(Findlay p.18)*.

- There should be professionally led mechanisms, as for instance through clinical audit, for ensuring that entries into medical case notes and nursing records are satisfactory both in terms of quantity and quality *(Findlay p.18)*.

- Steps should be taken to ensure that each member of the nursing management team from the Director of Nursing Services on the one hand to the supervising sister/charge nurses on the other knows precisely what are his/her role, responsibilities and lines of communication upwards and downwards *(Simpson p.12)*.

- In Ward 2 or any facility for the care of seriously disturbed patients, the admission of a patient who is not seriously disturbed because there is no other bed available should not occur; the operational policy for such facility should make it clear that this should not be permitted *(Simpson p.28)*.

- In Ward 2 or any intensive care facility at St. Edwards which may have 12 or more patients, there should normally be no less than four members of nursing staff on duty from the start of the night-shift until 11 pm. If such ward or facility admits male and female patients, include two women, one of whom should be a qualified nurse *(Simpson p.36)*.

- Because of the special nature of an intensive care facility, consideration should be given to taking such a facility out of the ordinary staff rota system and arranging that the sister/charge nurse in charge of such a facility, who as a result of the national clinical grading exercise has overall continuing responsibility for the ward, should have the specific duty of considering and deciding whether the staff numbers ordinarily provided for any shift are adequate. S/he should have the authority to call in extra staff or to require the attendance of a small number of staff (if e.g. patient numbers have declined) and, if appropriate after discussion, to vary working hours to meet demand *(Simpson p.36)*.

  Nursing management should
  - determine and agree an appropriate normal staffing establishment for any intensive care facility in the light of experience and expected workload;
  - ensure that sufficient additional staff can be provided to enable the sister/charge nurse in charge of such facility to discharge their responsibility;
  - have regular monthly meetings together with supervising sister/charge nurses from night and day at which past and future staff levels are reviewed *(Simpson p.36)*.

- Management and staff representatives should forthwith begin negotiations to enable rotation to be introduced as soon as possible between the night and day-shifts for the relatively small number of nursing staff, including nursing assistants, who work on any intensive care facility *(Simpson p.39)*.

- On Ward 2 or any other intensive care facility there should be in every week a multi-disciplinary meeting attended as far as possible by medical staff, other mental health professionals and representatives of the nursing staff at which should be discussed managerial, staff and procedural matters for the ward as a whole and matters relating to the care, treatment and security of individual patients. The sister/charge nurse in charge of the ward, if necessary in conjunction with the appropriate Clinical Nurse Managers, should be responsible for ensuring that, if possible, at least one member of the night staff is present at each meeting *(Simpson p.39)*.

- Because of the special need for good communication in any intensive care facility, such meetings should be minuted; and the minutes should be kept together in a readily accessible place known to all staff who work in the facility and should be circulated to each discipline. Consideration should be given to the provision of the services of a part-time ward clerk to any intensive care facility (this provision need only take up a relatively small number of hours per week) *(Simpson p.39)*.

- Staff from night and day-shifts be encouraged to attend ward meetings even if they take place outside their ordinary working hours; it should be made clear that staff will be paid or given hours in lieu for such attendance; staff should be informed when such meetings are to be held *(Simpson p.39)*.

- Those responsible for supervising and managing the nursing staff on any intensive care facility night and day, should have regular monthly management meetings (in addition to the ward-based meetings) to discuss nursing problems together *(Simpson p.39)*.

- Appropriate in-service training for qualified nursing staff and for nursing assistants in the use and understanding of the nursing process should be established as soon as possible. Attendance should be compulsory. Day staff and night staff should be encouraged to regard themselves as equal contributors to the formulation of care plans and to regard care plans as the property and province of all staff in equal measure. The nurses in charge of wards on days should be encouraged to talk to their counterparts on nights and vice versa so as to discuss any new care plans or modifications to care plans and to discuss problems in the implementation of care plans on a regular basis. The aim must be to produce care plans that are workable for days and nights; they may need expressly to make different provisions for day and for night *(Simpson p.43).*

- It should be made clear that the nurse in charge of any shift, but in particular a night-shift, if he or she finds that a care plan cannot be implemented, should make a plain entry in the nursing process to that effect *(Simpson p.43).*

- The nurse in charge on a night-shift, if on reading the care plans s/he believes that there may not be sufficient staff to put the care plans into effect, having regard to the condition of the patients, should be encouraged to contact his/her supervising sister/charge nurse to decide whether extra staff should be supplied, before, and not after, trouble develops *(Simpson p.43).*

- Care plans and modifications to care plans should be discussed as far as reasonably practicable with the doctor in charge of the patient. They should strive to achieve, as an ideal, the standard set out in the following quotation from an answer given in April 1989 by Mr. John Tait (Principal Nursing Officer, Department of Health), to the Select Committee on the Parliamentary Commissioner for Administration:
"I think it is important in formulating a care plan for any patient ... that there is joint consultation between doctors and nurses, that the nursing care plan dovetails into the medical prescription and that there is agreement between the doctors and nurses about the level of supervision required" (Simpson p.43).

- The key worker system should be extended to the night shift (although each member of the night-shift may have to be key worker for more patients than those who are key workers on the day-shift; this would not be an unfair burden) *(Simpson p.43).*

- An appropriate system for monitoring the use and understanding of the nursing process on the part of nursing staff should be formulated and put in effect by nursing management without delay *(Simpson p.43).*

- Consultations should be held as soon as possible, between nursing management and the education department and other bodies thought to have an interest, with a view to the finalisation of a document setting out clear and unambiguous definitions of levels of observation which are to be understood and acted upon by all staff involved, in any degree, in patient care. This document should be distributed to all relevant staff; it should make clear that all will be expected to absorb and apply its contents; managers should take steps to monitor the distribution and understanding of the document *(Simpson p.45).*

- Written policy or other document upon the method of conducting handovers should be produced as soon as possible, after consultation with all interested parties. Consideration should be given to the possibility of distinguishing between the requirements of an effective handover in a ward of seriously disturbed patients and the requirements elsewhere *(Simpson p.47).*

- In any intensive care facility, it would be appropriate to provide a handover period of no less than half-an-hour. We express one reservation to this recommendation. If at any time there is on such a facility only a very small number of patients, half-an-hour would not in fact be needed. But the difficulties of changing the handover time allowed in such a facility according to the number of patients could be substantial. If, for the sake of safety, half an hour were provided, it would give every opportunity to ensure a full and proper handover in an area in which it is necessary to be sure that a full and proper handover is taking place. If a full and proper handover were achieved more quickly, the spare time could doubtless be put to good use. Appropriate arrangements should be made for the monitoring of the effectiveness of handovers *(Simpson p.47).*

- An appropriate body involving management and the education department should meet regularly to decide upon the provision of appropriate in-service training courses, to select and encourage or, where apposite, even to compel staff to attend appropriate courses both internal and external *(Simpson p.50).*

- Consideration should be given to training or instruction upon the need to maintain, as far as possible, the levels of observation required by their patients' care plans even if attention is diverted by an incident involving one of their patients *(Simpson p.50).*

- It should be clarified that the nursing assistant is a full member of the nursing team in the delivery of care and in the translation of the care plan from paper to action; all nursing assistants must be given training in the importance and operation of the nursing process *(Simpson p.51).*

- There should be a pool or list of appropriately trained and experienced staff available for allocation to Ward 2 or any other intensive care facility when replacement staff are necessary *(Simpson p.52).*

- There should be a central register of clinical policy and guideline documents; the register should record which documents have been placed on which wards and when *(Simpson p.53).*

- Each clinical policy and guideline document should be drawn up with the active participation of staff in the operational way in which they apply and should record
  - a clear indication of its authors;
  - the date of its completion;
  - a specified date for review *(Simpson p.53).*

- An appropriate mechanism should be devised
  - to ensure that suitable policies or guideline documents exist for all operational areas;
  - to ensure that such documents are consistent throughout the hospital or Mental Health Unit as appropriate and are consistent with any relevant District or wider policies or guidelines;
  - to monitor the use of such documents in training *(Simpson p.53).*

- A file or folder containing all relevant policy and guideline documents should be maintained on each ward in a place which is readily accessible to all; so far as possible, it should be in the same place on each ward. There should be an index to each file or folder so that a nurse looking for guidance can see at a glance what is in the file or folder; and again, so far as possible, the index should be similarly structured in each ward *(Simpson p.53).*

- The putting into effect of annual reviews of performance, abilities and training needs for all staff, and a full review of communication throughout the structure of the Mental Health Unit with a view to the speedy development of more effective communication *(Simpson p.54).*

- An appropriate form of quality assurance should be incorporated into the system operated by the Mental Health Unit *(Simpson p.55).*

- Consultations between nursing management and consultants should take place with a view to arranging a more effective forum for discussion between them *(Simpson p.55)*.

- A representative or representatives of the District Health Authority should establish liaison with (local Regional Secure Unit) in order to discuss their respective roles in and to formulate a joint policy, within the terms of any regional policy, for the management of difficult-to-place disturbed patients *(Simpson p.59)*.

- Acute disturbed patients should not be cared for together with chronic disturbed patients. Acute seriously disturbed patients should, so far as possible, be nursed integrally with other patients *(Simpson p.119)*.

IN-PATIENT CARE - Treatment

- The Responsible Medical Officer must ensure that recorded case histories are both comprehensive and accurate and that case notes are regularly updated. Particular attention must be paid to the initial history and inadequacies rectified at the earliest opportunity *(Armstrong p.97)*.

- An assessment pursuant to s.2, MHA should be long and full enough to be able (as far as possible) to assess the risks to self and others if the section is discharged. This must include the risk of absconding *(Grey p.49)*.

- Such an assessment should include gathering as much information about the patient from as many sources as possible. If the patient has been transferred from prison, the probation service should be contacted to provide any relevant information and a check should be made of his antecedents for convictions involving violence *(Grey p.50)*.

- In respect of behaviour modification programmes and particularly in the absence of valid patient consent, a locally agreed procedure should be adopted in which the RMO should seek the advice of a suitably qualified person who is not a member of the clinical team responsible for the patient. This will normally be a psychologist, although some medical staff, social workers and nurses have received special training that equips them to supervise psychological procedures *(Mitchell p.175)*.

- Any member of staff who has been threatened or attacked by a patient should not be involved in taking an immediate decision to change that patient's treatment plan but should consult other members of the clinical team or even a second medical team *(Blackwood p.77)*.

- As part of the review of pharmacological management of patients, the Director of Medical Services should devise a hospital policy on measuring drug levels, introduce a clear policy on the administration of medication over BNF limits and initiate accurate monitoring of medication levels *(Blackwood p.77)*.

- The Hospital Advisory Committee (as the Managers defined in the Mental Health Act 1983) should ensure that, in line with the Code of Practice, a form is devised to be completed by the patient's RMO every time urgent treatment is given under s.62, Mental Health Act 1983. Managers should also monitor the use of urgent treatment (s.62) *(Blackwood p.77)*.

- Extreme caution should be taken when injecting struggling patients and, wherever possible, it should be avoided *(Blackwood p.77)*.

- Patient's written treatment plan should include an indication of to whom the Responsible Medical Officer function is delegated in the absence of the RMO *(Blackwood p.80)*.

- The administration of medication in a toilet is unacceptable *(Latham p.4)*.

- Strenuous efforts should be made to increase the engagement time of the residents and the amount of time spent off the wards *(Latham p.8)*.

- A comprehensive report should be drawn up on the use of psychology and remedial therapy and the facilities of the social education centre, clearly identifying any shortfalls in staffing or accommodation, and proposals should be made for rectifying the situation *(Latham p.8)*.

- A clinical review should be organised as a matter of urgency of those residents with repetitive behaviour disorders who may benefit from referral to psychologists *(Latham p.8)*.

- An appraisal should be made of the documentation currently held for each resident and rationalisation should take place *(Latham p.10)*.

- Each resident's records should contain information on the positive aspects of care in addition to recording illness and disturbed behaviour. The comprehensive needs of each resident should be recorded and, where these needs cannot be met, there should be a clear statement indicating the reasons why *(Latham p.10)*.

- The induction checklist used for student nurses should include reference to the Mental Health Act 1983 and the legal rights of the residents. It should be supplemented by clinical information on the residents' needs, likes, dislikes and strengths *(Latham p.10)*.

- Medical history on admission should be well and fully written and gathered afresh from original sources. Information should not be simply transferred from previous hospital records. The quality of the formulation of the patient's problems and preparation of a management plan should be of a high quality *(Ashworth p.239)*.

- When there is a change of RMO, all records relating to patients in their charge should be passed on to the newly arrived RMO and a full clinical handover should occur *(Ashworth p.256)*.

- Staff should receive regular training and refresher courses on the preparation and implementation of care plans. A system of clinical nursing audit should be implemented for monitoring the quality of care plans *(Ashworth p.260)*.

- Throughout their relatives' stay, families should be involved on a regular basis with their relatives' treatments *(Ashworth p.260)*.

- The Health Authority should encourage debate on the nature and treatment of mental illness particularly in relation to medication. High dosages of drugs need to be justified in the light of potential benefits weighed against the often very distressing side-effects. Patients' perceptions of side-effects need to be given due consideration by all *(Oxfordshire p.8)*.

- Opportunities should be created for more one to one therapeutic counselling of patients, and for care teams to obtain better understanding of patient's underlying personalities. Respect for the individual hidden within the patient must be maintained always *(Oxfordshire p.8)*.

- Present systems for the supervision and training of junior medical staff should be reviewed *(Shrodells p.9)*.

- The policy on prescribing over the telephone should be reviewed *(Barratt p.9)*.

- From the time of the first admission assessment, the Patient Care Teams should provide treatment and management plans, to include a programme of activities for all patients *(Watts p.25)*.

- Consideration should be given to the formulation of formal guidance upon the means by which and the circumstances in which communication between consultants who have dual responsibility for a patient's care should be maintained *(Simpson p.116)*.

- Consideration should be given to ensuring satisfactory arrangements for the "specialling of patients at risk" including the provision of the necessary resources. Where possible observation of patients requiring "specialling" should be by staff familiar with both the patient and the ward *(N.Lincolnshire vii)*.

- The nature and duration of observation required should always be made clear in the nursing records and care plans *(N.Lincolnshire p.vii)*.

- All relevant details relating to the administration of Electroconvulsive Therapy (ECT) should always be clearly recorded in a patient's medical records *(N.Lincolnshire p.viii)*.

- Guidelines should be issued to nursing staff concerning the recording of the administration of ECT. A review of documentation and forms concerning the use of ECT should be made in the light of relevant guidance *(N.Lincolnshire p.viii)*.

- Appropriate evaluation of care should be recorded in case notes. Entries by nursing staff in case notes should be always be signed and dated *(N.Lincolnshire p.xi)*.

- It is important to recognise that the responsibility for ensuring that an adequate care plan is available for each patient rests with the nurse in charge of the ward *(N.Lincolnshire p.xi)*.

- Changes in the legal status of patients should always be clearly recorded in the medical and nursing records *(N.Lincolnshire p.xii)*.

- The decision to administer heavy sedatives should be made by a doctor and not by nursing staff. The decision should be made at the time of the incident by a doctor in attendance on the ward who should be made fully aware of the extent of violence immediately preceding their attendance and of the quality and quantity of food recently consumed by the patient *(Martin p.15)*.

- Observation of a heavily sedated patient should be constant and should take place within the side room in which they are confined *(Martin p.15)*.

IN-PATIENT CARE - Physical health

- Special Hospitals Service Authority and the Mental Health Act Commission should consider producing guidelines on the lifestyle management of special hospital patients *(Blackwood p.79)*.

- All the targets set out in the Government's White Paper *Health of the Nation* should be adopted for special hospital patients and a named member of the clinical team should be responsible for applying the targets to each patient on an individual basis *(Blackwood p.79)*.

- Either the key worker or the health care assistant should have been available to have escorted Miss Latham to the City General Hospital and to have helped settle her back into the ward routine afterwards. It was a fairly unusual occurrence for a resident to undergo a barium meal examination and Miss Latham should have received careful monitoring upon her return to the ward *(Latham p.4)*.

- The leaving of a resident sitting on a toilet for more than a few minutes is unacceptable. While the Committee acknowledges the need to give residents as much privacy and dignity as possible, aids can be obtained for use within the toilet area to help support residents and it can certainly should not have been necessary to resort to any unauthorised form of restraint such as securing residents to the toilet cistern inlet pipe or handle. A toiletting programme had been written as part of a care review but it did not include the maximum length of time she was to be left on the toilet or any difficulties Miss Latham may have had in the toilet area which would have needed any form of mechanical support. The "hooking on process" was not documented but in any event this would have required approval by the Ethical Committee *(Latham p.4)*.

IN-PATIENT CARE - Control and Restraint

- Urgent action should be taken by the Director of Nursing Services to introduce training in the control of violent incidents without resorting in the first instance to physical restraint *(Blackwood p.78)*.

- Special Hospitals Service Authority should establish a research project to evaluate the efficacy of control and restraint procedures *(Blackwood p.78)*.

- Whenever Control and Restraint techniques are employed on a patient, there should be a post-incident review conducted by the full clinical team *(Blackwood p.78)*.

- As part of the review of the Control and Restraint Policy, a documented procedure should be approved and introduced to monitor the use of restraint *(Latham p.9)*.

- Forthwith, no mechanical restraint to be used at Ashworth Hospital *(Ashworth p.258)*.

- All nursing staff should be required to attend intensive courses in preventing violence *(Ashworth p.258)*.

- Control & Restraint should, whenever possible, be avoided; and to that end we recommend that the Special Hospital Service Authority determines a strategy which seeks to reduce the number of Control & Restraint interventions dramatically *(Ashworth p.258)*.

- When it has been necessary for any patient to be restrained, a physical examination should be carried out as soon as practicable *(Barratt p.9)*.

- All qualified nursing staff allocated to Ward 2 or any intensive care facility on a regular basis should, as soon as possible, attend either a training course in the management of violent and potentially violent behaviour or a control and restraint course or both. Consideration should be given to the provision of similar training courses to some nurses from other areas and in particular acute admission wards *(Simpson p.50)*.

- Proper training in physical control and restraint of patients should be given to all nursing staff *(Martin p.15)*.

IN-PATIENT CARE - Seclusion

- Trust board should supply the relevant Health Authority with a quarterly tally of episodes of seclusion with a brief explanation of each occasion *(NW London p.42)*.

- Hospital Management Team should undertake an urgent review of the suitability of rooms currently used to seclude patients *(Blackwood p.78)*

- Where a patient has been medicated while in seclusion, the nurse in charge should be responsible for checking the vital signs of the patient before the seclusion room is vacated, and the patient's vital signs should subsequently be monitored *(Blackwood p.78)*.

- Prior to entering a seclusion room, nursing staff should assess the mood and demeanour of the patient, and, unless circumstances demand entry, refrain from entering when it is concluded that such entry is likely to further disturb the patient. In any event, before entering the seclusion room, staff should inform the patient in a sensitive manner that they are about to enter the room *(Blackwood p.78)*.

- The number of nursing staff entering a seclusion room should always be kept to the minimum necessary to complete the task and in any event should never exceed 3 nurses in total *(Blackwood p.78)*.

- Seclusion should be phased out within the next 2 to 3 years *(Ashworth p.258)*.

- If seclusion of a patient does prove necessary, appropriate procedures (including the completion of relevant documentation) should be scrupulously observed *(N.Lincolnshire p.vii)*.

DEATH, INJURY, UNTOWARD INCIDENTS, COMPLAINTS AND INQUIRIES

- Those persons who conduct internal investigations and independent inquiries should always make early contact with family members, carers, people close to the patient and any victims to receive their views and information. They should keep them advised of progress and informed of the outcome of the Inquiry *(Sinclair p.76)*.

- As soon as possible after an incident involving a homicide by a patient (including an outpatient) in the care of the psychiatric services, there should be:
  (a) a clinical audit at immediate service level under the management of a clinician not involved in providing care for the patient, and
  (b) an internal inquiry. The treating clinical staff (including any Community Psychiatric Nurses who have been involved in the care of the patient) should be interviewed and detailed statements taken from them *(Hampshire p.70)*.

- Professional debriefing and access to counselling should be offered by the Health Authority to any member of the clinical team who expresses a wish to receive it *(Hampshire p.71)*.

- The immediate family of the patient should be invited at the earliest opportunity to discuss any matters relating to the care and treatment of the patient. Support should be offered to any member of the clinical team who agrees to meet with any such relative *(Hampshire p.71)*.

- Counselling or alternative support should be offered by the Health Authority to any member of the patient's family who expresses a need for such help *(Hampshire p.71)*.

- An Independent Inquiry must be set up at an early enough stage for the Panel to be able to start its investigations as soon as the outcome of any criminal proceedings is known *(Hampshire p.71)*.

- The consent of the patient to the release of all relevant records should be obtained at the earliest possible date and all such records should be obtained and delivered to the Inquiry Panel members in advance of the commencement of the Independent Inquiry *(Hampshire p.71)*.

- Any member of staff, or their managers, involved in direct work with a client, whose case is being investigated, should not be members of the internal review team. The role of these key staff would be to prepare reports and attend to give evidence as necessary *(Viner p.85)*.

- The Trust should establish serious incident policies and procedures, including details of the staff and personnel to be involved in any investigation and audit *(Viner p.85)*.

- Trust employees involved in managing reviews/audits should not be from the particular branch of the service concerned *(Viner p.85)*.

- The definition and classification of serious incidents needs to be developed *(Viner p.85)*.

- The processes of serious incident reviews/audits need to be re-evaluated to avoid a multiplicity of reviews *(Viner p.85)*.

- Internal reviews of practice following major untoward events should be conducted by a manager with no direct line management responsibility for the case in question *(Mitchell p.167)*.

- Employers, their legal advisers and insurers should find ways of helping their staff make direct personal contact with bereaved families, unless the families do not wish for this *(Mitchell p.221)*.

- A more direct, proactive and individual approach to the members of victims' families should be adopted by all agencies engaged in crisis support work following homicides and similar events *(Mitchell p.223)*.

- All authorities mandated to set up inquiries under NHS Executive Guidance HSG(94)27 should actively consider including in their terms of reference directions that families of victims should be given the opportunity to be present at any Inquiry into homicide, whether the Inquiry is held in public or private *(Mitchell p.223).*

- There should be greater clarity and explicitness in the guidance concerning the disclosure of documents to public inquiries *(Mitchell p.254).*

- The Rules of the Supreme Court - Order 38, rule 19(1), which authorise the Crown Office to issue a subpoena 'in aid of an inferior court or tribunal' should be reviewed by the Rules Committee to make it clear that non-statutory public inquiries, set up by central or local Government, qualify for subpoena powers *(Mitchell p.256).*

- Newham Social Services Department should undertake an audit of all service user files to ensure that personal information includes details of a next of kin and/or person to be contacted in case of illness, sudden death or other emergency *(Woodley p.129).*

- Although statutory authorities should be proactive in offering and providing support arrangements for bereaved or affected families in the case of untoward incidents, where the authority may be felt to be to blame we suggest that arrangements be in place to offer support by an independent person or organisation *(Woodley p.129).*

- All health and social services providers [should] have in place a plan of action for unexpected deaths and other untoward incidents *(Woodley p.129).*

- Where a placement has caused distress to neighbours, particularly where a violent incident has occurred, Housing Associations should determine their role in offering support and counselling *(Woodley p.130).*

- The Trust should ensure that there are formal procedures for debriefing staff in the event of a serious incident, whether the incident involves a current inpatient, outpatient or day patient or someone who has recently been discharged from inpatient, outpatient or day care *(Boland p.30).*

- It is essential that investigation of the death of a patient should always be conducted with expedition. The setting up of the inquiry should be instantaneous, with the composition of the team perhaps following a few days later. A report should have been in the hands of management, at most within six weeks. Once the report had been seen and, where necessary, acted upon by management, there is every reason why (the family) should have been supplied with a copy of the report and its recommendations *(The Falling Shadow p.129).*

- A standard preliminary exercise for all inquiry teams should be to compile an extended psychiatric and psycho-social summary, or chronology of the case, listing all significant events and all contacts between the patient and professionals and with independent sector services and organisations *(The Falling Shadow p.180).*

- Procedures should provide for the investigation of complaints objectively and separately from staff disciplinary proceedings and for the prompt and comprehensive written communication of the outcome of an investigation to complainants *(Thameside p.27).*

- All staff should be trained in understanding their role and function within the complaints system *(Thameside p.28 also Ashworth p.256).*

- When an internal Inquiry is carried out within a hospital or social services department, it is essential that not less than 2 members of the public are included on the panel to ensure that the Inquiry is as independent and objective as possible. Such members of the public should agree not to divulge any confidential information learned during the Inquiry *(Clunis p.124)*.

- Untoward events should continue to be discussed as a matter of course at the Trust Board meetings. In addition, any serious event should trigger a procedure agreed with the main purchasing authorities. An independent senior clinician or manager, not working in the Trust, is included on the team of those who investigate serious events. This process needs to be undertaken soon after an incident has taken place *(NW London p.42)*.

- Policies for checking equipment and for staff training in resuscitation need to be kept under close scrutiny, and to be uniform across the clinical units in the Trust *(NW London p.42)*.

- All staff should be given adequate training in all forms of resuscitation techniques appropriate to their discipline, and such training should be regularly updated. Part of the resuscitation procedure should include the immediate summoning of an ambulance *(Blackwood p.79)*.

- Clear policies and procedures should be developed for advising relatives of the death of a patient *(Blackwood p.79)*.

- Where relatives or friends are advised to come to the hospital, they should be advised to come by taxi and the cost should be met from hospital funds *(Blackwood p.79)*.

- Special Hospital staff accompanying the body of a patient to a general hospital should be encouraged to take all necessary steps to ensure that the minimum distress is caused to relatives of the patient *(Blackwood p.79)*.

- When a serious incident occurs individual professional reports should be collated and agreed as a definitive account of events and made available to all professionals concerned *(Inweh p.4)*.

- A written procedure should be introduced for dealing with untoward incidents and responding to emergency situations and a system should be developed for counselling staff after a serious incident *(Latham p.10)*.

- Training should be given to all members of staff who deal with relatives in the notification of a death *(Ashworth p.71)*.

- Referral to the police should be restricted to those cases where there has been a physical injury (of more than a minimal amount) or some other serious criminal offence *(Ashworth p.256)*.

- Each entry in the complaints register should give the name(s) of the complainant(s); the nature of the complaint and the name(s) of the person(s) about whom the complaint has been made. Possible development of a computerised database of complaints so that the number, type, location and severity can be monitored almost continuously *(Ashworth pp.256, 261)*.

- Referrals to the police should be contemporaneous with the complaint and investigation properly undertaken *(Ashworth p.256)*.

- If the time and effort in investigating thoroughly the complaints of loss of personal possessions, which do not involve theft, is prohibitive, it might be sensible to make an ex-gratia payment, with an express denial of legal liability *(Ashworth p.256).*

- Management and internal inquiry teams should be clearly instructed about the fundamental difference, on the one hand, between taking statements from witnesses, designed to ascertain the nature of the allegations and the personnel among staff and patients who can be identified as having been involved in the incidents to which the allegations relate, and, on the other hand, the finding of facts upon which others in authority can base their decisions. Some form of training is desirable and necessary in order that the stages of investigation are logically and clearly understood *(Ashworth p.256).*

- Before any other step in the complaints procedure is taken, (i.e. before any decision has been made as to whether an inquiry team is to be set up) an independent person must take a full written statement (a proof of evidence) from the patient *(Ashworth p.256).*

- Withdrawal of a complaint should never relieve management of a duty to explore the complaint fully and ensure that the withdrawal is in fact a true denial of the initial complaint *(Ashworth p.256).*

- Recognition of the importance of identifying one person to co-ordinate the appropriate response to the death of a patient, based on individual circumstances *(Ashworth p.259).*

- Special Hospital management should immediately inform the relatives on any death of a patient, that there will be an internal inquiry, irrespective of any inquest, and the inquiry report will be made available to them *(Ashworth p.259).*

- A pre-inquest meeting of all relevant staff, chaired by the Unit General Manager, should become part of the internal inquiry into a patient's death *(Ashworth p.259).*

- The General Manager should establish guidelines and procedures on the handling of serious and untoward incidents, which are not subject to the hospital's major incident procedure. Suitable training will be required for staff. In addition, an explicit procedure for the investigation of incidents must be established to include regular monitoring by those managers designated under the terms of the Mental Health Act 1983 *(Shrodells p.6).*

- The conduct of managers responsible for the service at the time of the incidents and nurses working in the unit should be investigated with a view to establishing whether disciplinary action is warranted. Where this is deemed to be so, and the individuals concerned are no longer employed by the Authority, their current employers and professional bodies should be informed of the outcome of the investigation. Should the nurses still be employed by the Health Authority, disciplinary action should follow the agreed procedures. The Regional Health Authority must decide whether the performance of senior medical staff warrants disciplinary action or referral to the appropriate professional body. The Chief Executive should report the performance of one locum doctor to the General Medical Council *(Shrodells p.9).*

- Guidelines and procedures for the systematic handling of complaints should be established *(Shrodells p.9).*

- It is essential that statements to the Press during an Inquiry should be jointly agreed between Health and Social services *(Barratt p.7).*

- Policy and procedure for reporting accidents and untoward incidents should include provision for the earliest practicable notification of all serious occurrences to appropriate senior officers *(Barratt p.9)*.

- Following an untoward incident which leads to police investigations, evidence should be collected by management as soon as possible, whilst seeking to maintain contact with the police to identify any areas where interests overlap and to avoid conflict with police inquiries during the pursuit of investigations by NHS managers *(Findlay p.19)*.

- The Clinical Nurse Manager for the acute area should carry out reviews of violent incidents on Ward 2 or any other intensive care facility either by reviewing each individually or by reviewing weekly the incidents occurring during the preceding week. It should be their duty, in discussion as necessary with other managers, to identify any necessary redeployment of resources and to establish and effect any necessary action *(Simpson p.31)*.

- An appropriate body should put into effect the original policy of the Violent Incidents Committee; it should meet no less frequently than once per month and should report to the UGM who should transmit information produced by such body to senior professionals in the Mental Health Unit. A representative of the staff of any intensive care facility should be a member of such body and should communicate the result of the body's work to the staff of that facility *(Simpson p.31)*.

- When medication is withdrawn from a patient who is disturbed or potentially violent or, in such a case, any other major change in treatment is put into effect, that step should be communicated to every member of the nursing staff who may have contact with that patient. Such communication should primarily be achieved by a clear entry in the nursing process. Nurses in charge of the ward at the beginning of a shift should have the express responsibility of communicating any such step which is recorded in the nursing process to the other nurses on their shift. If such a step has been discussed in a case conference or ward meeting, then the record of such discussion should also be available to the nurse in charge of the ward *(Simpson p.60)*.

- It should be made clear to all staff in an appropriate policy document that when anyone has been or may have been seriously injured, that person should not be left without the presence of a trained nurse or a doctor for any period, however short, in any circumstances *(Simpson p.95)*.

- Violent incident forms should only be completed by the nurse in charge of the ward on which the incident occurs or somebody in a senior position *(Simpson p.95)*.

- There should be a clear and plain policy document embodying the policy agreed with the police as to informing the family of a patient who has been the subject of an assault. Such policy should be produced and distributed forthwith. It could form part of a revision to the policy for the management of violent and potentially violent patients, or it could be a separate document. This policy document should also prescribe what steps staff must take to report to the UGM or other administrator an assault causing serious or significant injury, consistent with the policy decided upon as to reporting to the police so that a decision can be taken without delay as to who will inform the patient's family *(Simpson p.97)*.

- Pending national guidelines, a clear written local policy statement should be produced after consultation with the local police (preferably together with that dealing, by way of amendment to existing documents or in a separate document, with informing the family after a serious assault on a patient). We suggest that the following might form the basis of such a policy statement:

- ▲ In the case of any violent incident in which a patient has sustained really serious bodily harm at the hands of another person, that incident must be reported by the nurse in charge of the ward where it occurs or a nurse or nurse manager at a higher level as soon as possible to the UGM or, if the UGM is unavailable, to the next senior administrator in the unit (and at night to the designated on-call administrator) who must immediately report the incident to the appropriate police station and then inform the DGM of the action taken;
- ▲ In the case of a violent incident causing less serious but significant injury, the nurse in charge of the ward should have discussions with the UGM or an administrator appointed by the UGM for the purpose generally who, after consultation with the patient's consultant, should decide whether or not to report the incident to the police.
- ▲ In the case of minor injuries, the existing policy for violent incidents should be observed; reporting to the police should not arise *(Simpson p.100)*.

- There should be, in the case of any patient who is seriously disturbed for more than a short period, a strategic treatment plan specifically formulated for that individual patient; a clear statement of the diagnosis and of the treatment plan should be expressed both in the medical notes and in the nursing process *(Simpson p.116)*.

- The current procedure ... for handling serious untoward incidents, particularly involving patient care, should be reviewed as a matter of urgency. In particular the role of Unit and District Officers and of Health Authority Members, should be clarified *(N.Lincolnshire p.i)*.

- Independent clinical advice for any future fact-finding Inquiry ... should normally be obtained from outside the District *(N.Lincolnshire p.i)*.

- The Health Authority should ensure that the recommendations formulated by its Patient Services Panel viz.
  - ▲ a case conference should be held after each suicide or untoward incident;
  - ▲ a written report should be submitted to the Panel following the case conference,

  are implemented *(N.Lincolnshire p.i)*.

TRANSFER / LEAVE / CONDITIONAL DISCHARGE / DISCHARGE

- Discharge letters should contain the five key points outlined in "The Impact of a Hospital Audit on Psychiatrists' Letters to General Practitioners" (Shah and Pullen - Psychiatric Bulletin October 1995)
  (1) diagnosis, **(2)** treatment, **(3)** follow up arrangements, **(4)** prognosis and **(5)** a concise explanation of the condition *(Armstrong p.99)*.

- There should be some system of monitoring discharge letters written by Junior Medical Staff *(Armstrong p.99)*.

- There should be full consultation with nursing staff before any discharge of section and if possible also with any allocated Key Worker from the Mental Health Locality Team *(Grey p.50)*.

- No-one other than the RMO or another named Consultant can discharge any detention order under the MHA nor grant leave of absence to any compulsorily detained patient. We strongly recommend that this is clearly printed on the forms which need to be signed in order to discharge a section or grant leave of absence *(Grey p.50)*.

- A detention order should not be discharged immediately prior to transfer from a secure ward to an open ward. The section should remain at least long enough for the receiving ward to be able to assess how they need to manage the patient and the risk of absconding/risk to self and others in an open environment *(Grey p.50)*.

- There should be guidelines on good practice and procedures for the transfer and handover of responsibility for patients from one ward to another. These should include:
  - Identifying a named nurse for the patient on the receiving ward in advance of the transfer who will be "briefed" prior to the handover on all information relevant to ensure a continuity of care and assessment.
  - Having an agreed care plan to cover the transfer and the initial stages of the patient's stay on the new ward.
  - Agreement over the preferred legal status for the patient on transfer *(Grey p.50)*.

- A transfer from a secure to an open ward outside normal working hours should be avoided *(Grey p.50)*.

- The Nurse admitting the patient to the new ward should have available and read the nursing/medical notes prior to making their own admission assessment *(Grey p.51)*.

- The patient should be kept under special observation following transfer to an open ward until the staff are satisfied that it is no longer necessary *(Grey p.51)*.

- Any Key Worker who has been allocated (or a representative if not available) should attend all ward rounds involving their allocated patient and should be part of the decision making process concerning discharge of a section/transfer *(Grey p.51)*.

- The Discharge Summary should be completed by a doctor who knew the patient *(Grey p.51)*.

- A discharge from the hospital should not mean a discharge from the total resource of the mental health service. Once a patient is admitted to hospital they should become the responsibility of the linked catchment locality team until such time as they may be reallocated to a more appropriate team *(Grey p.51)*.

- A case must never be closed and a patient discharged from mental health care in ignorance of the patient's present health and welfare *(Grey p.51)*.

- All potential discharges 'Contrary to Medical Advice' should be discussed with the consultant psychiatrist responsible for their care or a senior deputy *(Doherty - N. Ireland p.77)*.

- All individuals who discharge themselves 'Contrary to Medical Advice' should be offered an early outpatient clinic review *(Doherty - N.Ireland p.77)*.

- There should be a recorded review of all patients who discharge themselves at the next multidisciplinary team meeting in order to formulate an aftercare plan and liaise with the relevant community services *(Doherty - N.Ireland p.77)*.

- In all instances where a voluntary patient is discharging him or herself "Contrary to Medical Advice", consideration should be given to the desirability of using powers to detain for assessment *(Doherty - N.Ireland p.83)*.

- When a sectioned patient on trial leave fails to cooperate with a plan of treatment s/he should be reassessed and, if necessary, recalled to hospital if there is no other way of making a speedy assessment *(Dalson p.15).*

- The discharge policy for the locked ward should be reviewed to ensure that there cannot be a rapid discharge of patients known to be at risk in the community. Placement in an open or rehabilitation ward should be considered. Failing this a period of leave under s.17, Mental Health Act 1983 should be used for detained patients *(Buchanan p.23).*

- Ad hoc arrangements for granting s.17 leave of absence should be reviewed to ensure procedures conform to guidance in the Mental Health Act Code of Practice *(S.Devon pp.47, 83).*

- Arrangements for the transfer of information contained in clinical notes between hospitals should be improved to satisfy the requirements of both transferring and receiving hospitals *(Kirkman pp.26, 38).*

- The clinicians responsible for making decisions about the transfer or discharge of patients should demonstrate that they have checked the original cause for the patient being in hospital, not only the changes in other aspects of the patient's behaviour *(Kirkman p.35).*

- All policies which regulate the discharge or transfer of patients should be written, regularly revised and their outcome subject to regular and automatic clinical audit by clinicians and management *(Kirkman p.35).*

- The Responsible Medical Officer should readily refer to a second consultant opinion before pressing for conditional discharge in doubtful patients. This would offset any good doctor's entirely desirable optimism on the patient's behalf, in contrast to the public's interest *(Kirkman p.35).*

- All bodies which are involved in making decisions about the discharge or transfer of mentally disordered offender detained patients but which are not in clinical contact should use figures gained from research and statistics and from predictive techniques to improve the quality of their judgements. These should supplement information gained from clinical sources *(Kirkman p.37).*

- Failure by officers delegated to receive documents on behalf of the managers to insist on the production of a written order who relied instead on Discharge Against Medical Advice Form *(Barratt p.6/7).*

- Insufficient consideration by RMO to provisions of s.17 leave (Barratt p.7). RMO's should be reminded that leave for a detained patient should be authorised in writing with appropriate conditions *(Barratt p.9).*

- Procedures should require the RMO to give a written order to the Managers of a Hospital before any patient detained under the Mental Health Act can be discharged from that section *(Barratt p.9).*

- As soon as it becomes evident that a patient is likely to discharge himself/herself against medical advice all professionals involved should be informed, and there should be a written procedure to ensure that, in whatever time is available, the best possible arrangements are made. The making of arrangements should wherever possible involve doctors (including GP's), nurses (including community psychiatric nurse), social worker and relatives *(Findlay p.18).*

- No patient who is or has recently been seriously disturbed should go out into the community, on leave or discharged, without a note as to the date on which and circumstances in which the patient leaves the hospital being made in the medical notes *(Simpson p.116)*.

- The status of patients upon leaving hospital (e.g. "on leave", discharged, outpatient, etc.) should always be clearly stated by medical staff, recorded and communicated to all parties involved *(N.Lincolnshire p.vi)*.

- Immediate telephone contact should be made with a patient's GP and other appropriate community support staff if the patient leaves hospital unexpectedly (including cases where patients take their own discharge) *(N.Lincolnshire p.vi)*.

- The procedure for the issue of "discharge notification" letters on the day of a patient's discharge should be reviewed to ensure that:-
  - ▲ the ward medical staff are directly involved with the completion of the "discharge notification";
  - ▲ the "discharge notification" should contain details of the patient's medication and follow-up arrangements;
  - ▲ copies of the "discharge notification" should be sent to the patient's GP and also any other community support staff directly involved with follow-up;
  - ▲ the "discharge notification" should normally be sent by first class mail (and not handed to the patient for onward transmission);
  - ▲ a copy of the "discharge notification" should be retained in the patient's medical records.

  The discharge summary should be completed by the medical staff as soon after discharge as possible *(N.Lincolnshire p.vi)*.

MISSING PATIENT / ABSENCE WITHOUT LEAVE

- The Missing Patients Procedure should be implemented in all cases where the patient leaves the ward and nothing is known of their whereabouts. No assumptions should be made that they will return to the ward. Managers should monitor the effectiveness and usage of the Missing Patients Procedure *(Grey p.51)*.

- Missing patient policy should include advice on contacting GP's *(Rooney pp.36,38)*.

MENTAL HEALTH REVIEW TRIBUNALS

- Efforts should be made to ensure that the medical members of tribunals dealing with restricted patients are forensic psychiatrists *(Mitchell p.136)*.

- The third category member of the Mental Health Review Tribunal should be named 'other relevant discipline' and the Lord Chancellor's list should include a number of psychologists *(Mitchell p.137)*.

- The medical member of the tribunal should expect the hospital to provide a set of summary documents with reports from the professionals involved in the multi-disciplinary teams responsible for the patient's care and treatment *(Mitchell p.139)*.

- Attention should be given to identifying and meeting more thoroughly the training needs of existing, as well as new Mental Health Review Tribunal members *(Mitchell p.246)*.

- Tribunal members should be informed about the clinical outcomes for patients following discharge decisions, and confidential retrospective reviews should be held in cases where patients re-offend seriously after discharge *(Mitchell p.246)*.

- A pending Mental Health Review Tribunal should not be a reason to discharge a section. The following developments are recommended:
  - If the patient is transferred to a new ward immediately or very shortly before the tribunal hearing, the reports for the tribunal should be prepared by the practitioners who know the patient best;
  - There should be regular training for all staff on MHRT procedures and requirements;
  - The Trust should invite the Mental Health Tribunal Office to join in a review of the working and the outcomes of recent tribunal hearings and procedures in Hackney Hospital, and draw up proposals for development, including proposals for discussion on the role of MHRT's. We recommend guidelines should be drawn up for the approach in future towards MHRT's *(Grey p.50)*.

- RMO's submitting medical reports to Mental Health Review Tribunals should make themselves available in person at the hearing wherever practicable *(Barratt p.9)*.

- The consultant psychiatrist responsible for a patient should attend a Tribunal hearing concerning that patient, and therefore every effort should be made for the Tribunal hearing to be arranged on a mutually convenient date *(Findlay p.17)*.

- A qualified nurse who is directly involved in a patient's care should always accompany the patient at a hearing of the Mental Health Review Tribunal *(Findlay p.17)*.

- When there is a change of consultant having responsibility for a patient during the period between the patient lodging an appeal to a Tribunal and the appeal being heard there needs to be effective liaison between the two consultants on the preparation of the medical report *(Findlay p.17)*.

- Reports prepared for Mental Health Review Tribunal hearings should routinely be exchanged, whenever possible before the hearing, between the professionals preparing the reports *(Findlay p.17)*.

HOUSING

- It is necessary for the individual housing associations which deal with general and special needs housing for vulnerable client groups, to have a clearer appreciation of the role and function of the responsible housing authorities. This will involve the establishment of clear written procedures and appropriate training for staff involved *(Viner p.39)*.

- Increased awareness of the routes which should be followed in dealing with housing applications by persons with mental health problems should be developed. This applies to both social services and health staff. This could be addressed by more formal guidelines and appropriate training *(Viner p.39)*.

- In relation to special needs housing, housing agencies should review their information and record-keeping systems wherever there is knowledge of mental health service involvement. This is to ensure that there is an adequate written record of transactions which take place. In a Care Programme Approach case, the lead agency should be provided with copies of all relevant documents and also the length of time records are kept should be re-evaluated *(Viner p.40)*.

- The role of the Housing Liaison Groups in relation to Special Needs Housing should be clearly specified and all relevant professionals should be advised of the Group's function in this area. Attendance of health professionals at these Groups, at operational level, should be reviewed to ensure that there is adequate input from the health services in this process *(Viner p.40)*.

- A high priority should be given to the development and maintenance of the database and the information contained in the database should be made available to all relevant professionals who become involved in the housing field. The existence of the database should be publicised, particularly to health keyworkers *(Viner p.40)*.

- Procedures should be established to deal with all housing applications received by housing associations. This should encompass referral to the social services department or to the relevant Community Mental Health Teams, and to the housing authority for assessment and prioritisation *(Viner p.41)*.

- Consideration should be given to establishing a common housing register *(Viner p.41)*.

- Bed and breakfast hotel accommodation should not be used for homeless people with mental health needs *(Woodley p.106)*.

- Where social work or health practitioners make a supporting application for ordinary housing in respect of people recovering from a severe mental illness who have a forensic history of violence, they must disclose this aspect in their report, together with a risk assessment giving explicit reasons why ordinary housing is considered appropriate. The report to the housing agency must identify the Care Programme Approach key worker or Community Care manager as a contact in the event of concerns *(Woodley p.106)*.

- The service users' permission must be sought for disclosure from health and social services records to housing agencies of information about themselves, and the content of and reasons for disclosure given to them *(Woodley p.106)*.

- Housing authorities and housing associations must have a policy on confidentiality which enables transmission of personal confidential information on the basis of 'need to know' for purposes of determining suitable housing allocation, and for the subsequent protection of service users, staff and members of the public *(Woodley p.106)*.

- The service user must be informed of how housing policy on confidentiality will operate. The housing policy must allow for access by service users to their own housing records *(Woodley p.106)*.

- The housing agency must notify the service user's key worker / care manager of the name of the housing officer who will have most contact with the service user, and of the housing management support role they perform. Thereafter the key worker / care manager must ensure that effective liaison is maintained with the housing officer *(Woodley p.106)*.

- The key worker / care manager, or housing officer, should review with a service user, who is socially isolated, their contact with neighbours. Where it appears that a neighbour has, or would be likely to offer a befriending role, that neighbour should be approached, and the identity of the key worker / care manager or housing officer made known as a contact in the event of concerns about the service user's well-being *(Woodley p.106)*.

- The Housing Department should, for all cases coming to their attention of people who are both homeless and severely mentally ill, consult with, take advice from and collaborate with the appropriate Social Services Department. Decisions regarding placement should be made jointly taking into account the opinion of the key worker. There is a need for exchange of information and provision of expert advice between Social Services Departments, statutory mental health providers and the Housing Department *(Newby p.153)*.

- Homeless people assessed as vulnerable by reason of mental illness should automatically be referred for assessment by social services unless this has already been carried out. The Department of the Environment should include this requirement in guidance to homeless persons units *(Newby p.154)*.

- Housing should be regarded as an integral part of a care plan by key workers and care managers *(Newby p.154)*.

- Providers of housing with care should take all reasonable steps to identify the needs of people referred to them, and satisfy themselves that they can meet these needs. They should ensure that their referral forms ask direct questions regarding all their criteria for acceptance and for exclusion. They should ask these questions of the individual referred, and of all the care agencies involved: crucial information may only be known to one agency *(Newby p.154)*.

- Housing associations and voluntary agencies providing housing with care should take all reasonable steps to meet the professional standards of care required by their residents. Such agencies should recognise that they are no longer meeting the needs of people who fall outside the mainstream of community care: they are providing the mainstream of community care *(Newby p.154)*.

- The Westminster Housing Department and its Medical Adviser, together with the Medical Practitioners and the Health Authorities in the borough should establish a formal mechanism through which they develop and keep under review the medical criteria and the application procedures for obtaining priority housing on medical grounds *(Boland p.31)*.

- Such criteria and procedures should accommodate the difficulties liable to arise with applications for housing priority which may be based on psychiatric, as opposed to physical, disorders *(Boland p.31)*.

- The criteria and procedures, together with the limitations on the total number of lettings available for applications made on medical grounds, should be publicised within the borough *(Boland p.31)*.

- The Policy and Procedures Group of the Housing Department should improve the scope and quality of the advice it provides to housing officers on how to implement policies and on the procedures that the Group lays down *(Boland p.31)*.

- The Housing Department should examine the nature and occasion of the guidance given by senior managers to junior housing officers in cases of particular complexity *(Boland p.31).*

- The Housing Department should, as part of service development, examine its procedures, publications, standard letters and other communications, internal and external, to ensure that they are clear, comprehensive and comprehensible *(Boland p.31).*

- After discharge, patients should be placed in appropriate supportive accommodation, staffed and resourced to deal with the patients needs and behaviour *(Buchanan p.23).*

- The Health Authority should investigate, together with the DSS and other agencies, possibilities for providing more "sheltered" types of accommodation with appropriate levels of support for mental health patients in the community, and more Community Psychiatric Nurses and Psychiatric Social Workers to increase after-care provision and back-up *(Oxfordshire p.2).*

- Where the clinical team which is responsible for the discharge and continuing care of a patient asks a housing association or department to provide accommodation for a "patient at risk", the advice of a specialist adviser in mental health should always be sought by the housing association. Patients at risk for these purposes are those who have been detained in Special Hospitals in the past, are to be followed up under s.117, or conditionally discharged restricted patients. If the housing association does not employ a specialist adviser in mental health itself, it should be put in touch with either the Social Services Department or another association which has one, for advice *(Kirkman p.35).*

- The specialist adviser should be invited to a predischarge multidisciplinary planning conference, with the patient's consent, and thereafter, without breaking confidentiality, should advise the housing association on the type of accommodation which is suitable and also what is not. Housing associations should be advised to choose housing for prospective tenants which takes into account the vulnerabilities and the special characteristics of the patients *(Kirkman p.36).*

- Consideration should be given in conjunction with social services to the introduction of a register of approved lodgings for former psychiatric patients, including an associated system of inspection *(N.Lincolnshire p.ii).*

RESIDENTIAL CARE

- Any establishment providing full-time and permanent care for severely mentally ill people will require the services and expertise of trained mental health professionals. Responsibility for this provision and for its specification lies both with the managers of the establishment and with the registration authority. In addition all employees require a programme of in-service training. The programme of in-service training for employed staff and for volunteers should be intensified and be better directed to the needs of the severely mentally ill and the staff caring for them. To be more specific, without implying their relative importance or the amount of time that should be spent on each, the following should be considered:
    - the signs and symptoms of major mental illness;
    - understanding and learning to talk with severely mentally ill people;
    - substance abuse and its management: alcohol and drugs;
    - treatment and management of mental illness: physical, psychological and social;
    - Mental Health Act and its application;

- ▲ Care Programme Approach: Supervision Registers; power of supervised discharge;
- ▲ Risk assessment;
- ▲ emergency assessment and admission procedures;
- ▲ record keeping *(Newby p.151)*.

- ■ These topics should be in addition to those, such as coping with violent episodes, which are already covered. There are undoubtedly members of staff of the statutory authorities who could teach and conduct seminars on the above subjects. It would be a valuable exercise in tripartite co-operation (voluntary agencies, social services and health) to organise and carry out such a programme. The staffing, funding and organisation of work of the statutory authorities should allow for such teaching and discussion to be seen as an essential activity directed towards improving the health of the people *(Newby p.152)*.

- ■ There should be developed an NVQ or similar qualification to provide a "core competence" for those working with the severely mentally ill in the community *(Newby p.152)*.

- ■ In addition to providing a core competence, there should be a second accredited level for those operating as key workers *(Newby p.152)*.

- ■ The registration authority (Department of Social Services) through its duly authorised arrangements for inspection (Social Services Inspectorate) should specify clearly and unequivocally the standards required for each individual residential home (whether it be a part of a larger organisation or not) in terms of buildings and their layout, amenities and equipment; type of resident and their number; number of staff on duty at any time, their experience and professional qualifications; in-service training needs. The authority has a duty to ensure that these specifications are both fully understood and comprehensively complied with. Every visit of the registration authority to the residential establishment should be recorded *(Newby p.152)*.

- ■ There is a clear need for 'haven-type' accommodation for those who cannot cope in the community *(Clunis p.122)*.

- ■ There is a clear need for a range of supervised accommodation for those who suffer from mental illness, from intensively staffed hostels with a high degree of nursing care, through warden staffed self contained units, to accommodation that is reserved for mentally ill people who can live more or less independently *(Clunis p.123)*.

- ■ The matching of an individual to proposed accommodation needs to be prepared more systematically. Whilst taking account of an individual's preference, accommodation should be carefully assessed in terms of the individual's needs as well as the "care culture" of the establishment, overall competence and experience of staff and staffing levels, the existing mix of residents and appropriateness of the physical accommodation *(Usoro p.16)*.

- ■ Staff in community residential accommodation catering for mentally ill people should receive relevant and appropriate information, advice and training in working with mentally ill people *(Usoro p.16)*.

- ■ The Care Manager should be aware of the format of record keeping in the home/hostel and have access to records by prior arrangement with the owner/carer *(Usoro p.17)*.

- ■ The Care Manager should agree with the owner/carer how relevant information will be passed on, either orally or by reference to the home's records *(Usoro p.17)*.

- In the Care Manager's preliminary review of accommodation s/he should seek to ascertain information on the background, age and mix of residents in a home *(Usoro p.17).*

- The home owner should receive clear guidelines on who to contact and how to obtain advice and support at all times and particularly out of hours *(Usoro p.17).*

- The contents of the application form for the hostel be reviewed by Kingston MIND and the question relating to 'life threatening behaviour' should be re-drafted to clarify its meaning, and, if answered in the affirmative, to include an accurate account of the behaviour *(Inweh p.5).*

- Kingston MIND should review staffing and security and take advice regarding the options available e.g. alarm systems to give greater protection to staff when working on their own *(Inweh p.12).*

- The use and availability of potentially dangerous kitchen or other implements in the hostel should be reviewed *(Inweh p.12).*

- Kingston MIND should consider the possibility of arranging for the regular psychiatric support for its hostel which we feel would be beneficial *(Inweh p.13).*

AFTERCARE - General

- The Trust should ensure that the Care Programme Approach is fully implemented in line with national guidance, that its implementation is fully audited using available audit tools, and that staff are fully trained to ensure that both the spirit and the letter of the Care Programme Approach are embraced and adopted *(Grey p.51).*

- That social services and district health authorities promote the involvement of voluntary organisations run by black and other ethnic minority groups in aftercare planning for inpatients from these communities *(Woodley p.109).*

- If discharge summaries are to be regarded as credible sources of information - and there is little point to them unless they can be so regarded - then they must be accurate, not only in their record of the immediate episodes of care, but also in their outline of the patient's historical perspective *(The Falling Shadow p.139).*

- Meetings to discuss the discharge of patients under the Care Programme Approach or via s.117, Mental Health Act 1983 should be attended by representatives of all disciplines involved in the care of the patient. In respect of mentally disordered offenders this should include representatives of the Police and the Probation Service when there has been contact with the patient in the past and social workers and Community Psychiatric Nurses in all cases *(Buchanan p.23).*

- A named worker should be allocated at the meeting to co-ordinate the care of the patient following discharge *(Buchanan p.23).*

- Multi-disciplinary involvement in discharge planning should be extended to the police and Probation Service where there is a likelihood of reoffending *(Buchanan p.24).*

- Insufficient attention has been given to s.117 aftercare procedures and the Care Programme Approach which must be addressed as matters of urgency *(S.Devon pp.47, 83)*.

- The aftercare needs of each individual patient must be assessed by health and social services before the patient is discharged into the community. Such assessment must take into account the patient's own wishes and choices *(Clunis p.110)*.

- A plan of care must be formulated for each individual patient, under the direction of the Consultant Psychiatrist under whose care the patient has been admitted *(Clunis p.110)*.

- The plan of care must fully consider and provide for the immediate and long term needs of the patient *(Clunis p.110)*.

- The plan must be formulated by all those who will afterwards be responsible for providing any part of the aftercare, so that the plan is made by a team of people who work in a variety of different fields. Such a team for convenience is called the multi-disciplinary team. The aftercare plan must be recorded in detail and a copy of the plan must be given to the patient and to all those who are to provide care *(Clunis p.110)*.

- Members of the multi-disciplinary team should be aware that aftercare is not provided by medication alone, although it is obviously a useful part of the armoury. There is always a need to help the patient come to terms with his illness and for the patient to have proper contact with those people who will be providing him with aftercare *(Clunis p.110)*.

- A keyworker must be agreed who will act to co-ordinate the care that has been planned by the multi-disciplinary team *(Clunis p.110)*.

- The aftercare which is provided must be properly co-ordinated and supervised; it is severely to the patient's detriment if each member of the team acts in isolation. The Consultant Psychiatrist and Care Manager from social services must together be responsible for supervising aftercare *(Clunis p.110)*.

- It is essential that each member of the team who is providing care for the patient responds effectively to signs and symptoms which suggest that the patient is likely to relapse. Help which can be given before a crisis develops is more beneficial to the patient than the care that can be provided once the patient is in crisis *(Clunis p.110)*.

- GP's should be informed of all aftercare plans *(Clunis p.128)*.

- Discharge summaries should be sent to GP's by fax or at the latest by post within 5 working days of discharge *(Clunis p.128)*.

- Ensure that the care programme approach is a regular part of clinical procedures *(NW London p.42)*.

- The Care Programme Approach should be implemented consistently throughout the service to an agreed timescale in line with Department of Health guidelines *(Usoro p.16)*.

- Arrangements should be made for communication of key information between all relevant parties involved in the care programme. The Care Manager, or another designated person, should be responsible for receiving and disseminating information to the various parties *(Usoro p.17)*.

- The Health Authority needs to look closely at the application of discharge and transfer policies and the comprehensiveness of care plans and, if necessary, construct a more formal framework to ensure that the movement of vulnerable patients between types of care or care teams is achieved in the most supportive manner possible *(Oxfordshire p.2)*.

- The policy of gradual and care introduction of patients such as these back into the community should be strictly adhered to, in spite of pressure on beds. They should not be discharged into isolated accommodation unless back-up can be provided on a consistent daily basis, at least in the early stages. The advisability of leaving such patients to make contact on their own initiative needs to be reviewed *(Oxfordshire p.3)*.

- The Care Group Manager, Mental Health, should ensure that there is an effective discharge procedure including effective arrangements for the after-care and discharge of all patients in accordance with the Care Programme Approach *(Shrodells p.8)*.

- Appropriate follow-up arrangements for patients should always be agreed before discharge and communicated to all concerned *(N.Lincolnshire p.vi)*.

AFTERCARE - Monitoring

- It is essential that the aftercare for patients is properly monitored by Health and Social Services *(Clunis p.111)*.

- Any area of unmet need which is identified by the multi-disciplinary team must be brought to the attention of the managers of the Health and Social Services *(Clunis p.111)*.

- In all cases covered by aftercare arrangements a regular, perhaps three monthly community care summary should be prepared by the lead officer responsible for aftercare in the community and communicated to worker; Community Psychiatric Nurse; the consultant; GP and to the officer in charge of any relevant residential and day unit *(Inweh p.11)*.

- A service register of all patients subject to after-care should be instituted with particular attention to the matters raised in paragraphs 29-46 of the Royal College of Psychiatrists publication (1991) 'Good medical practice in the aftercare of potentially violent or vulnerable patients discharged from in-patient psychiatric treatment' *(Inweh p.14)*.

AFTERCARE - Patient moving to another area

- The key workers should follow patients across Health and Social Services Board boundaries until responsibility is formally transferred to a local specialist team *(Doherty - N.Ireland p.81)*.

- When the patient moves from the district where he has previously been receiving care, responsibility for his aftercare should be formally transferred to the services responsible for his care in the district to which he moves *(Clunis p.110)*.

- Although Health and Social Services often have boundaries and catchment areas which do not overlap, proper co-operation between those who are providing care is likely to resolve any potential problems. Catchment areas should never be allowed to interfere with proper care in the community *(Clunis p.110)*.

AFTERCARE - s.117, Mental Health Act 1983 - General

- Any patient transferred to hospital under ss.47/49 should be seen as being subject to a full and comprehensive assessment of their health and social needs in accordance with the Care Programme Approach, Level 3 *(Grey p.49)*.

- District health authorities and local social services authorities should make it obligatory for their respective representatives to attend aftercare planning meetings pursuant to their duties under s.117, Mental Health Act 1983 (and in so doing facilitate such attendance) *(Woodley p.52)*.

- Kneesworth House Hospital should ascertain the availability of key personnel from district teams before convening statutory aftercare planning meetings *(Woodley p.52)*.

- The keyworker or a senior nurse on the ward familiar with the patient should always attend the s.117 meetings *(Buchanan p.23)*.

- The implications of discharge should be considered at s.117 meetings, particularly for patients known to be a risk to themselves or others or those with criminal records *(Buchanan p.23)*.

- The forms used for s.117 planning should be reviewed and expanded to reflect the decisions made, incorporating details of individual responsibilities for those involved in the aftercare and identifying the name of the keyworker *(Buchanan p.23)*.

- A new form should be designed for use in all s.117 aftercare cases, similar to other forms which are presently standardised under the Mental Health Act 1983 *(Clunis p.111)*.

- The form should record details of the plan that has been agreed, and should name the Consultant Psychiatrist, the Care Manager and the keyworker who together are responsible for the supervision and co-ordination of the plan *(Clunis p.111)*.

- Details of the signs and symptoms which suggest a likely relapse should be recorded as should details of the steps that the patient would like to be followed in the event of a relapse occurring. An assessment should be made as to whether the patient's propensity for violence presents any risk to his own health or safety or to the protection of the public *(Clunis p.111)*.

- Decisions and further plans that are made subsequently at s.117 review meetings, should be recorded on the form as should the decision to discharge the patient from s.117 aftercare *(Clunis p.111)*.

- The nominated keyworker in s.117 aftercare should always be a qualified and experienced Social Worker or Community Psychiatric Nurse *(Clunis p.112)*.

- A nationally based Register for patients subject to s.117 aftercare should be set up and lodged with the Mental Health Act Commission, where information which leads to ready identification of the patient would be stored, and which would indicate whence confidential information about the patient could be obtained *(Clunis p.112)*.

- GP's should always be invited to attend s.117 aftercare meetings and aftercare meetings for vulnerable or severely ill patients *(Clunis p.128)*.

- Policy and practices under s.117, Mental Health Act 1983 should be agreed and implemented without delay *(Inweh p.14)*.

- The content and layout of the local documentation re. s.117 aftercare should be revised and provision made for additionally recording:
  - ▲ specific comments about violence or other problems such as non-compliance with medication:
  - ▲ date(s) on which formal reviews will be undertaken;
  - ▲ termination of care under s.117, together with the reasons for such decision.

  The distribution of this form should be agreed and clearly marked on the form. Responsibility for distribution should be clearly delegated *(Inweh p.14)*.

AFTERCARE - s.117, Mental Health Act 1983 - Befriender/Advocate

- Every patient, subject to s.117 aftercare, should have a nominated relative, friend or volunteer to act as his befriender/advocate, unless the patient expressly states to the contrary *(Clunis p.113)*.

- Statutory Authorities and Voluntary Agencies working in the field of mental health should recruit, train and support members of the public who wish to be s.117 befrienders *(Clunis p.113)*.

- A copy of the current aftercare plan should be given to the befriender *(Clunis p.113)*.

AFTERCARE - s.117, Mental Health Act 1983 - Patient moving to another area

- Before a patient moves from the area where he is being cared for, a joint case conference should be held between those who are currently providing his aftercare and those who will be providing his aftercare in the future. Responsibility will remain with the original multi-disciplinary team unless and until s.117 aftercare is effectively transferred and a new s.117 form is completed by the new multi-disciplinary team *(Clunis p.113)*.

AFTERCARE - s.117, Mental Health Act 1983 - Monitoring

- The policy and procedures for the discharge of their duties under s.117, Mental Health Act 1983 should be reviewed to ensure that they have quality assurance monitoring in place to satisfy themselves that the individuals concerned are no longer in need of such aftercare services *(Woodley p.109)*.
- s.117 forms should be reviewed regularly by the Hospital Managers as defined under the Mental Health Act 1983 *(Clunis p.113)*.
- The Mental Health Act Commission should carry out external monitoring of s.117 forms on each statutory visit *(Clunis p.113)*.

SUPERVISED DISCHARGE ORDERS

- A patient who is detained for treatment under the Mental Health Act 1983 may be made the subject of a Supervised Discharge Order *(Clunis p.114)*.
- The Supervised Discharge Order should contain details of a plan of care which the patient and his Responsible Medical Officer have agreed *(Clunis p.115)*.
- If the Responsible Medical Officer considers that the patient has failed to comply with the plan, or that the patient's mental health is deteriorating, the patient may be recalled to hospital *(Clunis p.115)*.
- A Supervised Discharge Order shall be capable of renewal within 6 months of the Order being made and for 12 monthly periods thereafter, but only on the same grounds as the original Order was made *(Clunis p.115)*.
- Each renewal will be subject to the Mental Health Act 1983 appeal procedure *(Clunis p.115)*.
- The patient's Responsible Medical Officer, social worker and keyworker should be named in the Order as should the patient's relative or friend *(Clunis p.115)*.
- When the patient moves to another area those who are nominated in the Order should remain responsible for his care unless and until such care is properly transferred under the Order *(Clunis p.115)*.
- Supervised Discharge Orders should be lodged with and monitored by the Mental Health Act Commission *(Clunis p.115)*.

SPECIAL SUPERVISION GROUP

- Each supervision group patient should have a key worker, usually a specially trained community psychiatric nurse with a limited caseload and the facility to refer to other members of the team with special expertise *(Doherty - N.Ireland p.81)*.

- We endorse the recommendations of the Ritchie Report that caseloads of key workers working with seriously mentally ill people who are difficult to engage in services, must not be allowed to exceed a very limited number; we would estimate between eight and a dozen patients *(The Falling Shadow p.185)*.

- The Trust should give consideration to the establishment of a Supervision Register Team. It should be dedicated to provide support and an outreach service to people on the Register, particularly mentally disordered offenders *(Buchanan p.24)*.

- The resources necessary for the effective implementation of the Supervision Register and, where necessary, increasing such resources to reflect the demands of inner city levels of psychiatric morbidity. This should be reconsidered urgently if it is to effective *(Buchanan p.25)*.

- It is suggested that patients who suffer from a mental disorder and who are assessed by their Consultant Psychiatrist to require close supervision and support and who meet 2 of the following criteria would fall into that group:
  - ▲ patients who have been detained in hospital under the Mental Health Act 1983 on more than one occasion;
  - ▲ patients who have a history of violence or of persistent offending;
  - ▲ patients who have failed to respond to treatment from the general psychiatric services;
  - ▲ patients who are homeless.

  It is this Special Supervision Group whom we consider should be placed on the Supervision Register which was recently announced by the Secretary of State for Health *(Clunis pp.116/117)*.

- A nationally based Supervision Register for the Special Supervision Group should be set up, where information which leads to ready identification of the patient would be stored, and which would indicate from where confidential information about the patient could be obtained *(Clunis p.117)*.

- Every psychiatric service should identify patients as part of a Special Supervision Group and should provide a Specialist Team to supervise and support the group. New funding should be provided *(Clunis p.117)*.

- Every psychiatric service should appoint specialist Community Psychiatric Nurses to the team responsible for the Special Supervision Group whose only job is to supervise a very limited case load *(Clunis p.118)*.

- Community Psychiatric Nurses should follow patients across health boundary borders until responsibility is formerly transferred to another specialist team *(Clunis p.118)*.

- The National Health Service Executive should set up a panel to supervise inquiries commissioned under Health Service Guidelines HSG(94)27. The panel should:
  (I) be responsible for creating a register of those suitably qualified, both professionally and in their interpersonal skills, to sit on such inquiries and
  (ii) publish a recommended form of procedure and additional guidance designed to reduce delay and the stress caused to witnesses, particularly the relatives of the deceased and other victims, and to encourage cost-effectiveness *(Sinclair p.77).*

- Consideration should be given at the highest possible level to the possibility of giving inquiries the power to subpoena witnesses and documents *(Armstrong p.101).*

- The House of Lords' decision in *Secretary of State for the Home Department v. Oxford Regional Mental Health Review Tribunal* [1988] A. C. 120 should be reversed by law so as to allow a tribunal to adjourn an application in order to give time for a further examination of the patient's mental health before any decision to discharge is made *(Mitchell p.143).*

- Four general measures in respect of restricted patients should be considered by the Home Office:
  - ▲ C3 Division of the Home Office should act as a repository of information about the patient's index offence(s) *(Mitchell p.151);*
  - ▲ The procedures and practices of C3 Division could usefully be compared with Home Office practice in relation to Discretionary Lifer Panels *(Mitchell p.151);*
  - ▲ The notes for the Guidance of Social Supervisors should be reviewed and revised to take account of potential conflicts in the roles of social workers arising from changes in the Community Care, Mental Health and Criminal Justice legislation *(Mitchell p.167);*
  - ▲ The Case Worker Guide should be updated to require information not just from the RMO but from others who will bear responsibility for the after-care of the patient *(Mitchell p.154).*

- The Department of Health should draw together the existing fragmented policy guidance on the role of Local Authority and Health Services staff in the care and after-care of mentally ill people in an integrated document of guidance *(Mitchell p.167).*

- Given the need for close networking between many agencies and the establishment of supervision registers, some thought should be given by the Department of Health and the professional bodies to drawing on the best practice from child protection in developing an inter-agency approach to case management for mentally ill patients who are discharged into the community *(Mitchell p.168).*

- The 'Appropriate Adult' system in criminal justice should be re-examined with a view to extending its role *(Mitchell p.216).*

- The Secretary of State for Health should set in train a review of the Mental Health Review Tribunal system in the context of a review of the Mental Health Act 1983 *(Mitchell p.230).*

- The relevant Government departments should set a target date by which time all social supervisors of restricted patients will have acquired the competencies in forensic social work set out by CCETSW *(Mitchell p.241).*

- The Department of Health should ensure the funding of adequate numbers of training places for Clinical Psychologists *(Mitchell p.242).*

- The Government should consider establishing an independent committee to review the subject of the supply and dissemination of information within the services dealing with people in need of treatment, care and control *(Mitchell p.269).*

- The Secretary of State and the Royal College of General Practitioners and other appropriate GP organisations should consider the need for further guidance for GP's in dealing with potentially violent mentally disturbed patients in community care *(McFadden - Scotland p.27).*

- Compulsory supervision will be necessary from time to time using a supervised discharge order. This will require new legislation *(Doherty - N.Ireland p.81).*

- The Department of Health and Social Services (Northern Ireland) should review the Mental Health (NI) Order 1986 with the aim of introducing an additional category of mental disorder, namely severe personality disorder. This could follow the wording of s.3, Mental Health Act 1983 "... such treatment is likely to alleviate or prevent a deterioration of his condition" *(Doherty - N.Ireland p.83).*

- The Department of Health should give greater emphasis to preventative support work to children with parents with severe mental health problems, and commission and publish research which includes longitudinal studies, cultural variations and the effect of institutional racism *(Woodley p.21).*

- The Department of Health, Department of the Environment and Housing Corporation should make known the above recommendations to the agencies concerned - see HOUSING *(Woodley p.107).*

- The Government should increase the level of funding to the Social Fund for community care grants in areas of high need for mental health service users *(Woodley p.107).*

- The Benefits Agency should improve its performance in dealing with applications for community care grants (where otherwise delay affects an individual's ability to furnish and equip accommodation following the offer of rehousing, and where such delay incurs additional public expenditure, i.e. housing benefit on two tenancies) *(Woodley p.107).*

- The Department of Health should produce guidance, in consultation with public and voluntary bodies as well as with mental health service user representatives, on criteria for disclosure of personal confidential information concerning risk of violence where the public safety is the overriding consideration *(Woodley p.108).*

- The Department of Health, health authorities and social services authorities should recognise the need for and facilitate training in, on-going risk assessment and risk management for mental health practitioners in the context of multi-disciplinary working arrangements in the community *(Woodley p.108).*

- The Department of Health should harmonise guidance on s.117 Registers, proposed supervision registers, and the care programme approach with community care assessment and care management in respect of people who have a severe mental illness and their carers. Such guidance should include clarification of clinical, management and practitioner responsibilities, and the importance of choice by the service user in who their psychiatrist or key worker is to be for purposes of sustaining a therapeutic relationship *(Woodley p.109)*.

- The Department of Health, should, in issuing guidance, give recognition to disparities in information technology development throughout the health and social services *(Woodley p.109)*.

- The Department of Health, ... should give serious consideration to the need for 'bridging monies' to facilitate reprovision and the development of community based services for those with severe mental health needs *(Woodley p.162)*.

- The Department of Health should allocate additional funding as essential 'bridging monies' for purposes of local joint commissioning in areas facing the greatest obstacles to change and improvement in mental health provision. Such additional funding could be time-limited and reallocatable to other areas *(Woodley p.162)*.

- The Government should review the Personal Social Services Standard Spending Assessment in respect of community care for younger adults (16-64 years of age) *(Woodley p.163)*.

- The Department of Health should review its guidance to Local Authorities having responsibilities under the Registered Homes Act 1984 to ensure that:
    - ▲ The regulations should require the production of staff rotas to registration and inspection staff;
    - ▲ The regulations should require inspectors to check that the Care Programme Approach has been considered by registered homes;
    - ▲ The advice contained in Annexe 5 of Home Life is clarified to ensure that ambiguities in relation to staffing levels are removed *(Newby p.152)*.

- The Departments of Health and the Environment should clarify their responsibilities for funding housing for people with severe mental illness, and ensure that their funding arrangements are fully complementary. Adequate funds should be made available to house and provide care for all those with severe mental illness, including street homeless people, those with multiple problems, and those needing continuing long term care *(Newby p.154)*.

- Community care for the mentally ill and contributions towards that care coming from the voluntary sector ("the mixed economy") are both frequently expressed policies of the Government via the Department of Health. Government should specify standards of care and levels of professional qualifications and in-service training required by employed staff for the care of severely mentally ill people in the community and ensure that the resources are available to meet these standards *(Newby p.155)*.

- There is a real sense, communicated to us by staff of voluntary and statutory organisations and friends and relations of Jonathan Newby alike, that the loose structures of inadequate integration of separate services and meagre distribution of professional expertise appeared to have been sanctioned by Government in carrying out a new policy without adequate preparation and resourcing *(Newby p.155)*.

- The Department of Health should complete its review of confidentiality and information exchange between the various agencies involved in community care for people with mental illness, and disseminate clear guidelines widely *(Newby p.156)*.

- The Police, together with Social Services, should devise a system whereby when the Police are called to an address they would know whether the children are on the child protection register. We suggest this issue is taken up on a national basis by the Home Office and Department of Health *(Dalson p.12)*.

- An enhanced hospital order should be considered during future discussions on amendments to the Mental Health Act 1983. Such an order would allow longer term involuntary commitment of a patient under tightly defined criteria for treatable personality disorders. Although there is considerable disagreement about the treatability of such orders, the Panel accepts the view given by Dr Nigel Eastman that a spectrum of disorders exists from those who are wholly untreatable to those which are amenable to appropriate (probably psychological or psycho-therapeutic) treatments. Usually, treatment must take place in a secure setting where patients can feel a degree of safety, and which may take some years. Such an enhanced hospital order would require very careful drafting and controls including:
  - that such an order would only be used after other approaches to care had failed;
  - that a second specialist opinion was obtained on admission and subsequently at six month intervals;
  - that the patient would have the right to a Mental Health Review Tribunal to review the detention at regular intervals (normally six monthly);
  - that a multi-disciplinary review of the effectiveness of treatment be carried out at least annually.

  Such an order should encourage professional staff to consider offering treatments for periods of two or three years in the first instance subject to the criteria set out above (*Buchanan p.24)*.

- The availability of medium secure accommodation should be extended for patients with the mixture of mental disorder exemplified by Michael Buchanan. This recommendation is related to the recommendation on enhanced hospital orders. At present the special hospitals and regional secure units are highly reluctant to take patients with a diagnosis of personality disorder even with some form of overlaid but readily treatable psychotic component. Yet it is only by the availability of such long-term safe environments that patients such as Michael Buchanan will be able to settle to therapeutic regimes, including a range of psychological therapies, which will enable them to overcome the problems which 'created' the personality disorders in the first place. The Panel recognise that great care must be taken in deciding whether patients would require such long-term secure provision. Tight criteria would be required with very careful assessment and diagnosis. At present, however, significant barriers exist to providing patients such as Michael Buchanan with appropriate special hospital provision. This seems wholly unacceptable given public concerns *(Buchanan p.24)*.

- The Department of Health should determine, with the help of Directors of Social Services and others, how the confidentiality of mentally ill patients may be properly protected within the Care Programme Approach *(Clunis p.118)*.

- The Department of Health should publish the principles which community mental health services for the seriously mentally ill must follow, and declare minimum standards in manpower and facilities for all services to reach. These should be the basis of what the NHS Management Executive requires each Health Authority to commission for its community *(Clunis p.123)*.

- It is essential that the Department of Health sets up proper procedures for effective monitoring of psychiatric services in the community *(Clunis p.123)*.

- The Department of Health should institute a system to inspect community mental health services every 3 years, and to examine the results of health and social services annual joint reviews, so that national standards may be defined, maintained and improved upon *(Clunis p.124)*.

- The Home Office should publish a guide to interpreting Home Office Circular 66/90 re. Mentally Disordered Offenders in which clear advice is given as to when it is appropriate to charge someone who is mentally ill. Such advice should include guidance as to when medical opinion should be obtained, and to what matters should be taken into consideration, including the potential seriousness of the charge and the public interest *(Clunis p.126)*.

- Each body which is concerned with mentally abnormal offenders should, each year, report agreed measures which show the outcome of their decisions to the body to whom it is responsible. Reporting should be automatic, allowing performance to be judged and, if necessary corrected, and not left to fortuitous research. We believe that such checks on performance should apply to all such bodies without exception and include Mental Health Review Tribunals, the Advisory Committee on Restricted Patients, the decisions made about mentally disordered offenders by the Department of Health and the Home Office, the Special Hospitals Service Authority and the Regional Forensic Psychiatric Services *(Kirkman p.37)*.

- The Special Hospital Service Authority, Regional Secure Units and the Health and Home Office Departments should keep trying to find a better consensus with clinicians on the definition of treatability in personality disorder *(Kirkman p.37)*.

- Following consultation, the Department of Health should prepare guidance on placing patients, who have shown past evidence of dangerous behaviour, with housing associations and similar bodies *(Kirkman p.38)*.

- If a patient detained under s.2 of the Mental Health Act is transferred for good reasons between hospitals during the course of that period there should be a mechanism whereby an application can be made for the period of detention under s.2 to be extended so that 28 days can be available for assessment and treatment starting from the date of transfer between hospitals. There should also be a mechanism whereby the patient can appeal against such an extension. It is appreciated that this would require a change in the law *(Findlay p.17)*.

- The DHA and the RHA should press the Department of Health, the police and prosecuting authorities and the Home Office and any other professional organizations who can help to take steps to formulate national guidelines as to what assaults in psychiatric hospitals should be reported to the police *(Simpson p.100)*.